RESPIRATORY EMERGENCIES

A Practical Guide to Critical Care and
Life-Saving Strategies

Eric L. Oxley, MD, FCCM

Preface

In the realm of emergency and critical care, respiratory emergencies stand as one of the most dynamic and high-stakes challenges healthcare providers encounter. From acute exacerbations of asthma to catastrophic conditions such as pulmonary embolism and acute respiratory distress syndrome (ARDS), the ability to act decisively and with precision can mean the difference between life and death. Yet, despite their prevalence, respiratory emergencies often demand complex decision-making, interdisciplinary collaboration, and advanced technical skills that require continuous learning and mastery.

Respiratory Emergencies: A Practical Guide to Critical Care and Life-Saving Strategies was conceived to bridge the gap between foundational knowledge and real-world application. With healthcare environments growing increasingly complex and the demands on clinicians ever-rising, this book serves as a concise, evidence-based resource for medical professionals at all levels of expertise. Whether you are an experienced intensivist, an emergency physician, or a trainee encountering your first respiratory crisis, this guide is tailored to provide actionable insights, enhance diagnostic precision, and optimize patient outcomes.

As a physician specializing in critical care and emergency medicine, I have witnessed firsthand the transformative impact of timely interventions in respiratory crises. These experiences have informed my commitment to creating a resource that not only imparts technical knowledge but also emphasizes practical application. This book synthesizes the latest advances in diagnostic tools, therapeutic strategies, and life-support techniques, ensuring it remains a relevant and indispensable tool in the ever-evolving field of respiratory care.

Acknowledgments

This book is the culmination of years of clinical practice, research, and collaboration with colleagues who share an unwavering commitment to excellence in patient care. I extend my gratitude to the many mentors, peers, and trainees who have inspired me throughout my career. Their insights and experiences have shaped the content and approach of this guide. I also thank the patients whose resilience and courage continue to be a source of profound learning and inspiration.

Purpose and Scope

This book is designed to provide a comprehensive overview of the assessment, diagnosis, and management of respiratory emergencies. It is structured to address both the theoretical underpinnings and the practical aspects of care, offering clinicians a dual perspective that is both deep and broad. Each chapter incorporates case studies, clinical pearls, and evidence-based recommendations to guide readers through complex decision-making processes.

The scope of this guide extends across a wide spectrum of respiratory emergencies, from acute infections and obstructive airway diseases to life-threatening complications such as hemoptysis, pneumothorax, and ARDS. Recognizing that respiratory emergencies rarely occur in isolation, the book also emphasizes the multidisciplinary nature of care, exploring collaborative strategies that engage intensivists, emergency physicians, respiratory therapists, and other allied healthcare professionals.

Key Features

Practical Frameworks: A step-by-step approach to diagnosing and managing respiratory emergencies, tailored to real-world clinical settings.

Evidence-Based Insights: Integration of the latest research and clinical guidelines to support informed decision-making.

Case-Based Learning: Scenarios drawn from actual clinical practice to illustrate challenges and solutions in the management of respiratory crises.

Advanced Techniques: Detailed discussions of cutting-edge interventions, including bronchial artery embolization, extracorporeal membrane oxygenation (ECMO), and mechanical ventilation strategies.

Multidisciplinary Focus: Guidance on fostering teamwork and collaboration in high-pressure situations.

Final Thoughts

As you embark on this journey through Respiratory Emergencies: A Practical Guide to Critical Care and Life-Saving Strategies, I invite you to approach each chapter with an open mind and a critical eye. The management of respiratory emergencies is as much an art as it is a science, requiring both rigorous knowledge and adaptive thinking. My hope is that this book will not only enhance your clinical skills but also deepen your appreciation for the complexities and rewards of caring for patients in their most vulnerable moments.

Let us advance together, armed with the knowledge and compassion necessary to save lives and improve outcomes in the ever-challenging field of respiratory care.

Eric L. Oxley, MD, FCCM

Preface
Acknowledgements
Purpose and Scope
Key Features
Table of Contents
List of Abbreviations

Table of contents

Chapter 1: Introduction to Respiratory Emergencies

1. Overview of Respiratory Emergencies
   - Definition and scope
   - Common scenarios in healthcare settings

2. The Importance of Respiratory Emergencies
   - Role of the respiratory system in homeostasis
   - Consequences of respiratory failure
   - Urgency and impact on patient outcomes

3. Common Causes of Respiratory Emergencies

- Acute infections and trauma
- Chronic conditions and exacerbations
- Pulmonary embolism and other critical conditions

4. Challenges in Managing Respiratory Emergencies
- Variability in clinical presentation
- Subtle symptoms vs. critical escalation
- Complexities of respiratory interventions

5. The Multidisciplinary Approach
- Role of emergency physicians, intensivists, and respiratory therapists
- Importance of teamwork in patient management

6. Book Structure and Approach
- Clinical assessment and diagnostic tools
- Management strategies for respiratory crises
- Case studies and practical scenarios

7. Conclusion

- Importance of skill and decision-making in emergencies
- How this book equips healthcare providers for better outcomes

Chapter 2: Upper Respiratory Tract Emergencies

1. Introduction to Upper Respiratory Emergencies
- Overview of the anatomical region and functional significance.
- Common presentations: emergent vs. non-emergent cases.

2. Triage and Initial Assessment
- Identifying life-threatening conditions.
- Key clinical signs and initial examination.

3. Upper Airway Obstruction: Causes and Management
- Physiological and mechanical causes.
- Initial and advanced airway stabilization techniques.

4. Diagnostic Tools
- Role of endoscopy, imaging, and laboratory tests in assessment.

5. Foreign Body Airway Obstruction
- Clinical features and management strategies for partial and complete obstruction.

6. Trauma-Induced Upper Airway Injuries
- Blunt trauma: mechanisms, pathophysiology, and clinical presentation.
- Penetrating trauma: diagnosis and treatment protocols.

7. Thermal and Chemical Airway Burns
- Pathophysiology and clinical features.
- Management strategies for airway compromise and burns.

8. Radiological Features of Adult Epiglottitis
- Key imaging signs: thumb sign, vallecula sign, and prevertebral swelling.

Chapter 3: Asthma

- Legionella species
- Staphylococcus aureus

4. Clinical Investigations
- Imaging Techniques
- Chest X-ray (CXR)
- Computed Tomography (CT)
- Lung Ultrasound
- Laboratory Tests
- Full Blood Count (FBC)
- Urea, Electrolytes, and Liver Function Tests
- Blood Gas Testing and Inflammatory Markers
- Microbiological Testing
- Sputum and Blood Cultures
- Urinary Antigen Tests

5. Severity Assessment
- Scoring Systems
- Pneumonia Severity Index (PSI)
- CURB-65
- SMART-COP and CORB

6. Management
- Antibiotic Therapy
- Empiric Treatment Recommendations
- Considerations for Drug-Resistant Pathogens
- Adherence to Guidelines
- British Thoracic Society (BTS) Guidelines
- IDSA/ATS Recommendations

7. Special Considerations
- Elderly Patients and Comorbidities
- Resource-Limited Settings

8. Conclusion
- Optimizing Diagnostic and Treatment Approaches
- Importance of Guideline Adaptation to Local Contexts

Chapter 5: Influenza and Emerging Respiratory Infections

1. Introduction

- Overview of influenza as a global health concern
- Impact on healthcare systems and society

2. Microbiological Classification
    - Types of influenza viruses (A, B, C)
    - Subtypes and lineages (H and N classification)
    - Role of surface proteins in viral replication and targeting

3. Epidemiology
    - Seasonal influenza trends
    - Antigenic drift and antigenic shift
    - Historical pandemics and their global impact

4. Avian and Other Zoonotic Influenzas
    - Transmission dynamics in zoonotic strains
    - Public health implications of H5N1, H7N9, and swine flu

5. Incubation Period and Infectivity

- Contagiousness and virus survival on surfaces
- Risk factors for nosocomial transmission

6. Clinical Features
- Common symptoms and diagnostic challenges
- Severity spectrum across different populations

7. Complications
- Pneumonia (viral, bacterial, mixed)
- Systemic effects: cardiac, neurological, and muscular complications
- Differential diagnosis considerations

8. Clinical Investigations
- Laboratory markers (WBC, CRP)
- Imaging findings (X-ray and advanced modalities)

9. Influenza Preparedness in Healthcare Settings
- Infection control protocols

- Role of vaccination among healthcare personnel

10. Screening and Triage
    - Identifying influenza-like illnesses
    - Risk stratification and isolation measures

11. Managing Unsafe Practices and Aerosolization
    - Guidelines for nebulization and aerosol-generating procedures
    - Use of negative pressure rooms and PPE

12. Role of Flu Clinics in Preparedness
    - Establishing and managing flu clinics
    - Coordination between healthcare facilities

13. PPE and Antiviral Medication Supply
    - Stockpiling and allocation during outbreaks
    - State-level policies for healthcare worker protection

Chapter 6: Chronic Obstructive Pulmonary Disease (COPD)

1. Introduction
   - Overview of COPD as a leading global health challenge.
   - Pathophysiology and progression of persistent airflow limitation.
   - Impact of acute exacerbations on patient outcomes and healthcare systems.

2. Epidemiology
   - Global prevalence and projections.
   - Regional statistics, including data from Australia and New Zealand.

3. Aetiology and Pathogenesis
   - Role of smoking, genetic predispositions, and environmental factors.
   - Pathological mechanisms: inflammation, fibrosis, and structural changes.
   - Associated comorbidities like bronchiectasis and their clinical significance.

4. Clinical Features
- Gradual progression and common symptoms.
- Differentiation between stable COPD and acute exacerbations.
- Importance of patient history and baseline condition.

5. Diagnostic Approach
- Key investigations
- Role of arterial and venous blood gasses in acute settings.

6. Classification and Management of COPD
- Staging severity: mild, moderate, and severe COPD.
- Stepwise therapeutic interventions tailored to disease stage.
- Preventative measures

7. Management of Acute Exacerbations in the Emergency Department

- Immediate goals: diagnosis, severity assessment, and stabilization.
- Treatment strategies: bronchodilators, corticosteroids, and antibiotics.

8. Oxygen Therapy
- Principles of controlled oxygen delivery.
- Risks of hyperoxic hypercapnia and strategies to avoid complications.

9. Non-Invasive Ventilation (NIV)
- Indications, benefits, and limitations of NIV in acute respiratory failure.
- Comparison of CPAP vs. BiPAP and their clinical applications.

10. Invasive Ventilation
- Criteria for intubation and mechanical ventilation.
- Risks and considerations for critically ill COPD patients.

11. Long-Term Management Strategies

- Role of pulmonary rehabilitation and long-acting therapies.
- Nutritional considerations and management of systemic effects.

12. Future Directions and Research in COPD Management
    - Emerging therapies and innovations in patient care.
    - Addressing global disparities in COPD treatment access.

13. Summary and Key Takeaways
    - Essential points for clinical practice and ongoing patient management.

Chapter 7: Pneumothorax

1. Introduction
    - Definition and Types of Pneumothorax
    - Incidence and Delay in Medical Attention

2. Etiology and Contributing Factors

- Spontaneous Pneumothorax: Primary vs. Secondary
- Risk Factors
- Primary Spontaneous Pneumothorax (PSP)
- Secondary Spontaneous Pneumothorax (SSP)
- Genetic Disorders
- Iatrogenic and Traumatic Causes

3. Pathophysiology and Complications
   - Mechanisms of Air Leakage
   - Tension Pneumothorax: Pathogenesis and Clinical Impact

4. Clinical Presentation
   - Symptoms
   - PSP: Mild Symptoms, Sudden Onset
   - SSP: Severe Dyspnea and Associated Features
   - Physical Examination Findings

5. Diagnostic Considerations
   - Imaging Modalities

- Chest X-ray (CXR)
- Computed Tomography (CT)
- Ultrasound in Critical Settings
- Laboratory Investigations

6. Management Strategies
- General Principles
- Oxygen Therapy
- Emergency Decompression for Tension Pneumothorax
- Conservative Management
- Observation and Monitoring
- Invasive Interventions
- Simple Aspiration
- Chest Tube Drainage

7. Emerging Evidence and Future Directions
- Advancements in Less Invasive Techniques
- Ongoing Trials and Guideline Refinement

8. Conclusion
- Tailored Management for Optimal Outcomes

- Importance of Early Recognition and Smoking Cessation

Chapter 8: Pleural Effusion

1. Introduction
   - Definition and overview of pleural effusion.
   - Importance of identifying the underlying cause.
   - Diagnostic tools and techniques.

2. Pathogenesis and Pathophysiology
   - Normal pleural fluid dynamics.
   - Mechanisms leading to effusion formation.
   - Categories of pleural effusion: transudative, exudative, and lymphatic.

4. Etiology
   - Transudative Causes: Common and uncommon conditions.
   - Exudative Causes: Infectious, malignant, inflammatory, and iatrogenic factors.

5. Classification Using Light's Criteria
- Biochemical parameters to differentiate transudates and exudates.

6. Clinical Presentation and Evaluation
- History and Symptoms: Common presentations and systemic indicators.
- Physical Examination: Respiratory changes, auscultation, and percussion findings.

7. Diagnostic Investigations
- Imaging: Role of chest X-rays, ultrasound, and CT in diagnosis.
- Thoracentesis: Biochemical, microbiological, and cytological analyses.
- Additional Tests: Specialized markers for tuberculosis, chylothorax, and other conditions.

8. Conclusion
- Systematic approach to evaluation and management.

- Importance of Light's criteria in guiding diagnostics and treatment.
- Role of advanced imaging and fluid analysis in effective management.

Chapter 9: Haemoptysis

1. Introduction
   - Definition and clinical significance
   - Spectrum of haemoptysis: From mild to massive
   - Life-threatening implications of massive haemoptysis

2. Aetiology
   - Common causes of haemoptysis
   - Cases with no identifiable cause

3. Clinical Features
   - Differentiating haemoptysis from haematemesis and upper airway bleeding
   - Key symptoms and patient history considerations

4. Diagnostic Investigations
- Chest X-ray findings and limitations
- Role of high-resolution CT and CT pulmonary angiography
- Diagnostic value of bronchoscopy
- Laboratory tests and adjunct investigations

5. Treatment Approaches
- Non-Massive Haemoptysis
- Outpatient management and follow-up
- Massive Haemoptysis
- Airway, Breathing, Circulation (ABC) prioritization
- Emergency imaging and oxygenation strategies

6. Advanced Interventions
- Intubation techniques and challenges
- Circulation stabilization and hemostatic measures
- Bronchial artery embolization
- Rigid versus flexible bronchoscopy
- Surgical interventions

7. Additional Measures
- Endobronchial tamponade and topical treatments
- Management of specific causes

8. Conclusion
- Integrated diagnostic and therapeutic approaches
- Multidisciplinary management for optimal outcomes

List of Abbreviations

ABC: Airway, Breathing, Circulation

ATDs: Antithyroid Drugs

CT: Computed Tomography

CXR: Chest X-Ray

ETT: Endotracheal Tube

FCCM: Fellow of the College of Critical Care Medicine

HRCT: High-Resolution Computed Tomography

MRI: Magnetic Resonance Imaging

O$_2$: Oxygen

PHC: Primary Health Care

RAI: Radioactive Iodine

TB: Tuberculosis

Chapter 1
Introduction to Respiratory Emergencies

Respiratory emergencies are some of the most critical and time-sensitive medical conditions encountered in healthcare settings. Whether in the emergency department, intensive care unit, or during transport to a hospital, the ability to quickly identify, diagnose, and manage respiratory crises is a fundamental skill for all healthcare providers. These emergencies, ranging from acute asthma attacks to life-threatening conditions like acute respiratory distress syndrome (ARDS) and massive hemoptysis, require swift and precise interventions to prevent morbidity and mortality.

In Respiratory Emergencies: A Comprehensive Guide to Critical Care and Life-Saving Strategies, the aim is to provide healthcare professionals with a detailed, practical guide to effectively managing these urgent situations. This chapter serves as the foundation for understanding the critical role of respiratory emergencies in modern medicine and introduces the core concepts that will be explored throughout the book.

The Importance of Respiratory Emergencies

The respiratory system plays an essential role in maintaining homeostasis by ensuring efficient gas exchange between the lungs and the bloodstream. When the respiratory system falters—whether due to obstruction, restriction, or failure—the consequences can be immediate and severe, leading to hypoxia, acidosis, or even death if not treated promptly. The urgency of these conditions, coupled with the complexity of diagnosis and treatment, makes them a major focus for clinicians in the emergency and critical care environments.

Respiratory emergencies can be triggered by a variety of factors, including acute infections, trauma, asthma exacerbations, chronic obstructive pulmonary disease (COPD) flare-ups, pulmonary embolism, and massive bleeding, among others. These conditions not only require rapid assessment and intervention but also demand a multidisciplinary approach involving respiratory therapists, intensivists, emergency physicians, and other healthcare specialists. Each of these professionals must work in concert to provide life-saving care and improve patient outcomes.

Challenges in Managing Respiratory Emergencies

One of the primary challenges in managing respiratory emergencies is the variability of clinical presentation. While some patients may exhibit clear signs of distress, others may present with subtle symptoms that can quickly escalate into critical conditions. For example, a patient with acute asthma may initially appear mildly short of breath, but if untreated, could rapidly progress to respiratory failure. Similarly, conditions like pulmonary embolism or tension pneumothorax can present with nonspecific symptoms that require clinicians to be vigilant and thorough in their diagnostic approach.

The complexity of respiratory interventions is another significant challenge. From securing an airway in a patient with massive upper airway swelling to managing mechanical ventilation in patients with ARDS, clinicians must be proficient in a wide range of technical skills. This book will guide healthcare providers through these challenges by offering evidence-based protocols and practical tips for managing the full spectrum of respiratory emergencies.

Book Structure and Approach

In the following chapters, we will explore the key areas of respiratory emergencies, beginning with a detailed look at clinical assessment and diagnosis. You will learn how to effectively evaluate patients presenting with respiratory distress, utilizing diagnostic tools such as imaging, blood gas analysis, and pulmonary function testing. The book will then move into the management strategies for common and complex respiratory emergencies, emphasizing life-saving interventions such as mechanical ventilation, pharmacologic treatments, and advanced procedures like bronchial artery embolization and extracorporeal membrane oxygenation (ECMO).

Throughout the book, each chapter is designed to build upon the previous one, with case studies, practical scenarios, and expert commentary to guide your understanding. By the end of this book, you will be well-equipped to respond confidently and competently to respiratory emergencies, armed with both theoretical knowledge and practical, hands-on strategies.

Conclusion

Respiratory emergencies demand the highest level of clinical skill and rapid decision-making. This book is intended to serve as an indispensable resource for healthcare professionals, providing a clear and structured approach to managing these time-sensitive conditions. Whether you are a seasoned critical care physician or a resident in training, Respiratory Emergencies: A Comprehensive Guide to Critical Care and Life-Saving Strategies will help you navigate the complexities of respiratory crises, improve your diagnostic accuracy, and refine your intervention techniques to save lives and improve patient outcomes.

Chapter 2
Upper respiratory tract

Key points

1. Prioritizing the airway, breathing, and circulation (ABCs) is critical before addressing the history, examination, or specific management of upper airway obstruction.

2. Direct laryngoscopy serves as a valuable tool for both diagnosing and managing upper airway obstruction.

3. Chest thrusts and back blows are effective first-aid measures for relieving ,foreign body obstructions in the upper airway.
As
4. Acute viral respiratory infections frequently prompt medical consultations, and the

inappropriate prescription of antibiotics remains a significant challenge.

5. Although uncommon, bacterial infections and abscesses can compromise the upper airway and require prompt evaluation.

6. Diagnosing laryngeal and tracheal injuries from blunt trauma necessitates a high level of vigilance, particularly with potential cervical spine involvement.

7. Adult supraglottitis is becoming more prevalent, often presenting with nonspecific symptoms. However, invasive airway interventions are rarely required.

Comprehensive Overview of Upper Respiratory Tract Emergencies

The upper respiratory tract, spanning from the mouth and nose to the carina, represents a relatively small anatomical region of immense functional importance. While most cases presenting with upper respiratory complaints are non-life-threatening, certain conditions necessitate urgent assessment and intervention to avert airway compromise. Immediate protection of the airway and stabilization of vital functions (Airway, Breathing, Circulation—ABCs) supersede detailed history-taking, examination, or ancillary investigations.

Key Emergency and Non-Emergency Presentations

Emergent presentations, such as airway compromise from trauma, infection, or allergic reactions, demand immediate action to secure the airway. Non-urgent cases include facial swelling not affecting the airway, mild sore throats in stable patients, or chronic complaints without recent exacerbation. Common non-emergent conditions include pharyngitis and tonsillitis, which frequently appear in both pediatric and adult emergency scenarios.

Triage and Initial Assessment

Accurate triage is pivotal for differentiating life-threatening conditions from less critical issues. Key clinical signs of airway obstruction include:

Respiratory Symptoms: Dyspnea, stridor, altered voice, or dysphagia.

Increased Work of Breathing: Intercostal retractions, nasal flaring, or fatigue.

Late Indicators: Cyanosis and altered mental status.

Assessment begins with evaluating the general appearance, vital signs (temperature, respiratory rate, oxygen saturation), and localized findings, such as mucosal swelling or lymphadenopathy. The examination should adapt to the patient's presenting complaint and findings.

Upper Airway Obstruction: Causes and Management

Upper airway obstruction may arise acutely or insidiously and can result from physiological or mechanical causes, such as:

1. Physiological Causes: Decreased consciousness due to head injury, stroke, or metabolic disturbances.

2. Mechanical Causes:

Intrinsic: Foreign bodies or angioedema.

Wall-based: Tracheomalacia or trauma.

Extrinsic: Ludwig's angina or external compression.

Management begins with securing the airway, often through basic maneuvers like chin lifts or advanced interventions such as endotracheal intubation or surgical airways. The approach depends on the nature of the obstruction, with care taken not to worsen incomplete obstructions.

Diagnostic Tools

Investigations should follow stabilization and are guided by clinical findings:

Endoscopy: Direct laryngoscopy provides a definitive assessment, allowing removal of foreign bodies or securing an airway.

Imaging: Lateral neck X-rays or CT scans can identify masses, foreign bodies, or trauma-related injuries, though airway patency must be ensured before imaging.

Laboratory Tests: Blood gasses, cultures, and a complete blood count may offer additional diagnostic clues but are secondary to initial airway management.

Foreign Body Airway Obstruction

Foreign bodies in the airway present unique challenges, often related to an altered consciousness state or anatomical predisposition. Management depends on the severity of obstruction:

Incomplete Obstruction: Utilize conservative measures such as laryngoscopy or careful removal.

Complete Obstruction: Conscious patients may benefit from back blows or chest thrusts, while unconscious patients may require direct laryngoscopy, intubation, or surgical airway interventions.

Trauma-Induced Upper Airway Injuries

Blunt or penetrating trauma to the neck can result in airway obstruction. Mechanisms include direct blows, "clothesline" injuries, or hyperextension from sudden deceleration. Injuries may range from minor hematomas to cricotracheal separation, often accompanied by cervical spine damage.

Clinical Features and Investigations:

Suspect injury in cases of aphonia, stridor, or deformities.

Imaging and endoscopy should be conducted in stable patients to guide management.

Treatment and Emergency Interventions

Primary treatment focuses on airway stabilization using methods ranging from simple maneuvers to surgical options. While techniques like cricothyrotomy are rarely needed, familiarity with their application is essential. Subsequent management addresses the underlying pathology, guided by findings from endoscopy, imaging, and laboratory results.

By adhering to these protocols, healthcare providers can effectively manage upper respiratory emergencies, minimizing morbidity and ensuring prompt resolution of critical conditions.

Blunt Trauma to the Airway: A Detailed Overview

Incidence and Challenges in Diagnosis
Laryngotracheal injuries caused by blunt trauma are rare, accounting for approximately 0.3% of all trauma cases seen in emergency settings. The increasing recognition of these injuries may partly explain the rising reported incidence. Anatomically, the upper airway benefits from natural protection due to the larynx's mobility, the trachea's compressibility, and the shielding effects of the head and mandible. However, diagnosing these injuries can be challenging

since external examinations may appear normal, and other significant head or chest injuries can obscure symptoms.

Mechanisms of Injury
Common mechanisms include:

Clothes-line injuries: Cyclists or riders colliding with fences or cables.

Direct trauma: Impact from assaults, sports equipment, or industrial accidents.

Hanging incidents: Neck trauma and airway obstruction from ligature-related suicide attempts.

Dashboard injuries: Occurring in unrestrained passengers during vehicle deceleration, leading to neck hyperextension and laryngeal compression between the cervical spine and dashboard.

Pathophysiology

Frequent injuries include vertical fractures of the thyroid cartilage. Fractures of the hyoid bone or cricoid cartilage, ruptures of the cricothyroid ligament or vocal cords, arytenoid dislocation, and even complete cricotracheal transection can occur. Up to 50% of individuals with significant blunt airway trauma concurrently sustain cervical spine injuries.

Clinical Presentation

Suspected injuries should be evaluated in patients presenting with:

Voice changes, such as aphonia or hoarseness.

Breathing difficulties, including stridor or dyspnea.

Dysphagia.

Patients may present with complete airway obstruction or deteriorate rapidly upon arrival. Visible signs might be minimal or include laryngeal tenderness, deformity, or subcutaneous emphysema. Associated head, chest, or cervical spine injuries are common and warrant thorough assessment.

Investigations

Endoscopy: Flexible laryngoscopy or bronchoscopy is essential and should be performed in an operating room, prepared for potential surgical intervention.

Imaging:

X-rays: Lateral neck views can assess airway patency and identify subcutaneous emphysema or fractures. Elevation of the hyoid bone suggests cricotracheal separation.

CT Scans: These are superior for evaluating the extent of injuries to the airway, cervical spine, and surrounding structures, performed only after patient stabilization.

Classification of Injury Severity

Table 6.1.1 summarizes the grading of blunt laryngeal injuries based on endoscopic and radiological findings:

Grade I: Minor hematoma without fracture.

Grade II: Edema, minor mucosal disruption, or non-displaced fractures.

Grade III: Severe edema, exposed cartilage, or immobile structures.

Management

Airway Stabilization: Immediate management focuses on securing the airway while protecting the cervical spine. Fiberoptic bronchoscopic intubation minimizes complications such as false tracheal lumen creation or laryngeal disruption. Emergency tracheostomy may be necessary, ideally performed in the operating room.

Cricothyrotomy is avoided due to distorted anatomy.

Surgical Intervention: Indications for surgery include airway obstruction necessitating tracheostomy, uncontrolled subcutaneous emphysema, extensive mucosal lacerations with exposed cartilage, or displaced fractures. Early involvement of otolaryngology specialists is critical.

Prognosis

Mortality rates vary by injury site, ranging from 11% for isolated thyroid cartilage fractures to 50% for cricoid cartilage, bronchial, or intrathoracic tracheal injuries. Asphyxiation is the leading cause of mortality. Long-term complications may include persistent voice changes and difficulty swallowing.

Penetrating Trauma to the Airway

Mechanisms and Clinical Features

Penetrating injuries are typically caused by assaults, accidents during sports or industrial activities, or complications from malignancies or radiation therapy. Key signs include hoarseness, stridor, subcutaneous emphysema, and haemoptysis. Such injuries often coexist with damage to major vessels or pulmonary structures, necessitating prompt surgical management for hemorrhage control and airway stabilization.

Investigations and Treatment

The approach mirrors that of blunt trauma, emphasizing airway management and early surgical consultation.

Thermal and Chemical Airway Burns

Pathophysiology and Features

Thermal burns can result in airway compromise due to facial and neck swelling, laryngeal edema, or circumferential neck burns. Smoke inhalation, affecting 25% of burn victims, often leads to bronchospasm and impaired gas exchange. Chemical burns caused by inhaled or ingested caustic substances present similarly.

Management

Prompt intubation is critical in cases of stridor or hoarseness to prevent airway obstruction from progressive edema. Endoscopy and imaging guide further management.

Radiological Features of Adult Epiglottitis: Detailed Analysis

Key Radiological Signs and Measurements

1. Thumb Sign

This classic radiological finding reflects edema of the epiglottis, which normally has a leaf-like appearance.

The swollen epiglottis appears as a rounded, thumb-like shadow on imaging.

Diagnostic measurement: The width of the epiglottis in healthy adults is typically less than one-third of the anteroposterior width of the C4 vertebra. In adult epiglottitis, this width exceeds 9 mm, confirming significant inflammation.

2. Vallecula Sign

Progressive swelling of the epiglottis leads to a reduction or obliteration of the vallecula, the air pocket located between the tongue base and the epiglottis.

Normally well-defined, this space becomes narrowed or absent due to edema.

3. Aryepiglottic Fold and Arytenoid Swelling

Inflammatory changes result in the swelling of the aryepiglottic folds and arytenoids, contributing to airway narrowing.

4. Loss of Vallecular Air Space

The vallecular air space is no longer visible on imaging, indicating severe inflammation.

5. Prevertebral Soft Tissue Swelling

Measurement: The thickness of the prevertebral soft tissue should not exceed 50% of the anteroposterior width of C4. An increase beyond this suggests edema.

6. Hypopharyngeal Airway Widening

Diagnostic ratio: Normally, the hypopharyngeal airway width to the anteroposterior width of C4 should be less than 1.5. A higher ratio may indicate airway compromise secondary to inflammation.

Management of Adult Epiglottitis

1. Antibiotic Therapy

Broad-spectrum antibiotics targeting likely pathogens, including Haemophilus influenzae type b (Hib), Streptococcus pneumoniae, β-hemolytic streptococci, and Staphylococcus aureus, are essential.

Recommended agents include third-generation cephalosporins (e.g., ceftriaxone or cefotaxime). In cases with methicillin-resistant S. aureus (MRSA) concerns, alternatives like clindamycin are effective.

2. Steroids and Adrenaline

The utility of systemic steroids and nebulizer or parenteral adrenaline (epinephrine) in managing airway edema remains controversial. These agents may be considered on a case-by-case basis to reduce inflammation and improve airway patency.

3. Airway Management

Most adults respond to conservative treatment without requiring advanced airway intervention, such as intubation or tracheostomy.

Areas of Controversy

Antibiotic Standardization: Establishing clear protocols for antibiotic selection in adult pharyngitis and epiglottitis.

Role of Advanced Airway Techniques: The indications for intubation and adjunct therapies, including steroids and adrenaline, lack consensus.

Ultrasound Utility: The role of point-of-care ultrasound (POCUS) in diagnosing supraglottitis is emerging but requires further validation.

Evidence-Based Insights

Changing Trends: Research highlights shifting patterns in epiglottitis presentation and outcomes in the post-vaccine intervention Outcomes**: Systematic reviews suggest improved mortality rates and reduced airway intervention frequency with early recognition and management .

References

1. Alcaide, A. L., & Bisno, A. L. (2006). Pharyngitis and epiglottitis. Infectious Disease Clinics of North America, 21(3), 449–469.

2. Tamir, S. O., Marom, T., Barbalat, I., et al. (2015). Trends in adult supraglottitis: A

changing landscape. European Archives of Oto-Rhino-Laryngology, 272(4), 929–935.

3. Chroboczek, T., Cour, M., Hernu, R., et al. (2015). Outcomes in critically ill adults with acute epiglottitis: A retrospective cohort study. PLoS ONE, 10(5), e0125736. https://doi.org/10.1371/journal.pone.0125736

4. Solomon, P., Weisbrod, M., Irish, J. C., & Gullane, P. J. (1998). Adult epiglottitis: Clinical experience at the Toronto Hospital. Journal of Otolaryngology, 27(6), 332.

5. Ng, H. L., Sin, L. M., Li, M. F., et al. (2008). Acute epiglottitis in adults: A retrospective analysis of 106 cases in Hong Kong. Emergency Medicine Journal, 25(5), 253–255.

6. Abdalla, C. (2012). Acute epiglottitis: Current trends in diagnosis and management. Saudi Journal of Anaesthesia, 6(3), 279–281.

7. Marx, J. T., Blaivas, M., & Adhikari, S. (2014). The application of airway and thoracic ultrasound in clinical practice. Ultrasound Clinics, 9(4), 211–216.

8. Dore, L., Periyanayagam, U., McCarthy, D., & Courtney, D. (2012). Epiglottitis in adults: Mortality and airway intervention trends in the post-vaccine era. Annals of Emergency Medicine, 60(4), S64.

Chapter 3
Asthma

Key Points:

1. Global Impact: Asthma represents a significant global health burden, contributing to considerable morbidity and mortality rates worldwide.

2. Pathophysiology: The condition is marked by episodic bronchoconstriction and wheezing triggered by various stimuli.

3. Risk Factors for Severe Asthma: Individuals with the following characteristics are at heightened risk of life-threatening asthma episodes:

History of severe asthma attacks.

Previous admission to an intensive care unit (ICU) requiring mechanical ventilation.

Use of three or more categories of asthma medications.

Frequent use of β-agonist inhalers.

Multiple emergency department visits within the past year.

Recent (within six months) use of oral corticosteroids.

Behavioral or psychosocial contributors, including non-adherence to treatment plans, obesity, and mental health disorders.

4. Attack Severity: Asthma exacerbations range from mild to life-threatening and can escalate rapidly, sometimes within minutes.

5. Diagnostic Indicators: The severity of an asthma attack is effectively assessed through clinical evaluation, bedside pulmonary function tests, and pulse oximetry.

6. Core Treatments: Standard management involves administering oxygen, β2-adrenergic agents, and corticosteroids.

7. Criteria for Hospitalization: Hospital admission is recommended when:

Pretreatment peak expiratory flow rate (PEFR) or forced expiratory volume in 1 second (FEV1) is below 25% of the predicted value.

Post-treatment levels remain under 60% of the predicted value.

8. Environmental Triggers: "Thunderstorm asthma" is an uncommon phenomenon in which environmental factors induce asthma attacks, even in individuals without a prior asthma diagnosis.

Introduction

Asthma represents a substantial global health issue, contributing to significant levels of illness and death. Its prevalence varies worldwide, with regions like Australasia, New Zealand, and the United Kingdom reporting higher rates, affecting approximately 20% of children and 10% of adults. Many patients seek emergency department (ED) care when standard treatments fail to manage symptoms effectively. Asthma exacerbations can range from mild to life-threatening, necessitating immediate therapeutic intervention in emergency settings.

Other reasons for visiting EDs include running out of medication, experiencing symptoms after a symptom-free interval, or seeking a second opinion on asthma management. For such cases, ED care focuses on patient education, symptom management, and referral to appropriate long-term care providers.

Epidemiology

The Global Initiative for Asthma estimates that over 300 million individuals worldwide are affected by asthma. Regions like Australasia, the UK, and North America exhibit higher prevalence compared to the Middle East and parts of Asia. Severe cases are notably more common in Australasia. Geographic differences may be influenced by factors such as ethnicity, urban versus rural living environments, and air pollution. Epidemiological research suggests that asthma prevalence and severity are gradually increasing globally.

Aetiology, Pathophysiology, and Pathology

Asthma is characterized by airway hyper-reactivity and inflammation, leading to episodic, reversible bronchoconstriction triggered by various stimuli. It is a multifaceted, immune-mediated condition with a strong genetic predisposition, though no single gene has been conclusively linked to the disease. Instead, asthma is believed to have a polygenic basis, which explains its diverse clinical manifestations.

Triggers such as allergens, viral respiratory infections, pollutants, occupational exposures, emotions, exercise, and certain medications (e.g., aspirin and beta-blockers) initiate an exaggerated inflammatory response. This response activates cells like mast cells, eosinophils, basophils, Th2 cells, and natural killer cells, which release primary mediators (e.g., histamine) and secondary mediators (e.g., leukotrienes and prostaglandins). These mediators cause bronchoconstriction, increased vascular permeability (edema), and excessive mucus production.

Pathophysiological effects of acute asthma include:

Increased physiological dead space.

Respiratory muscle fatigue.

Intrinsic positive end-expiratory pressure due to hyperventilation and air trapping.

Thunderstorm Asthma

Thunderstorm asthma is an uncommon phenomenon triggered by specific types of storms. These storms lift grass pollen into the atmosphere, where the pollen absorbs moisture, ruptures, and releases microscopic allergen particles. These particles can be inhaled deeply, causing irritation and severe asthma symptoms. This event typically occurs during late spring or early summer when pollen levels peak.

People at increased risk include those with asthma, seasonal hay fever, or grass pollen allergies. However, individuals without known risk factors may also experience severe symptoms.

Clinical Assessment

Objectives of clinical assessment:

1. Confirm asthma diagnosis.

2. Evaluate severity.

3. Identify complications.

History:
Asthma presents as episodic shortness of breath, often accompanied by wheezing, chest tightness, and coughing, with symptoms worsening at night. Attacks may progress gradually or rapidly. Atypical presentations include persistent cough or reduced exercise tolerance.

Risk factors for life-threatening asthma include:

Previous ICU admissions requiring ventilation.

Dependence on multiple asthma medications.

Frequent ED visits within a year.

Recent use of oral corticosteroids.

Behavioral and psychosocial factors, such as medication non-compliance, psychiatric conditions, or socioeconomic stressors, may also increase risk.

Examination:

The severity of asthma influences physical findings, ranging from mild wheezing to respiratory failure. Severe asthma may present with:

Inability to speak normally.

Accessory muscle use.

Silent chest on auscultation.

Altered consciousness.

Oxygen saturation below 92%.

Clinical Investigations

Mild to Moderate Asthma:

Perform pulmonary function tests, such as PEFR or FEV1.

Chest X-rays are only required if complications like pneumothorax or pneumonia are suspected.

Severe or Life-Threatening Asthma:

Assess PEFR or FEV1 if feasible.

Conduct chest X-rays and arterial blood gas analysis for oxygen saturation below 92% or signs of respiratory fatigue.

Emerging evidence suggests venous blood gas analysis may reliably screen for hypercarbia and acidosis, reducing the need for arterial sampling.

Treatment

Emergency asthma management is guided by severity and Principles include:

Ensuring adequate oxygenation.

Reversing bronchospasm.

Minimizing inflammation.

Mild Asthma:

Administer salbutamol via MDI with spacer or nebulizer.

Consider oral corticosteroids if needed.

Moderate Asthma:

Repeat salbutamol as needed.

Add ipratropium bromide for poor response.

Prescribe systemic corticosteroids for 5–10 days.

Severe Asthma:

Initiate management in a resuscitation area with continuous monitoring.

Provide oxygen and escalate therapy as required.

Patients showing significant improvement after initial treatment may be discharged with corticosteroids and inhaled steroids. Those with persistent symptoms require further observation or intensive care.

Magnesium Sulfate in Acute Asthma Management

Magnesium sulfate is believed to exert bronchodilatory and anti-inflammatory effects. A Cochrane review indicates that a single dose of intravenous magnesium sulfate improves lung function and reduces hospital admissions in adults with acute asthma unresponsive to oxygen, nebulized short-acting β2-agonists, and intravenous corticosteroids. However, data is insufficient to establish its efficacy across different severity levels. Current guidelines recommend administering a single dose of intravenous magnesium sulfate (10 mmol over 20–30 minutes) for:

Acute severe asthma unresponsive to inhaled therapy

Life-threatening asthma

Ventilatory Support Strategies

Non-Invasive Ventilation (NIV):
For patients with adequate consciousness and airway protective reflexes, NIV can be considered to avoid endotracheal intubation. NIV reduces airway resistance, promotes bronchodilation, prevents atelectasis, decreases respiratory workload, and mitigates the cardiovascular effects of intrapleural and intrathoracic pressure changes. While it does not independently improve gas exchange, case studies show rapid pCO_2 correction and significant short-term improvement within an average of five hours. Compared to intubation, NIV is associated with fewer adverse events. Although there are no definitive guidelines, a trial of closely monitored NIV in appropriate patients is reasonable.

Mechanical Ventilation:
If NIV fails or is unsuitable, endotracheal intubation is necessary. Ketamine, due to its bronchodilatory properties, is the preferred

induction agent. Ventilation must be cautiously managed to avoid severe air trapping, which can cause elevated intrathoracic pressure and cardiovascular compromise. Recommended parameters include:

Ventilation rate: 6–8 breaths/min

Low tidal volumes

Prolonged expiratory phases
Permissive hypercapnia is acceptable if adequate oxygenation is maintained, reducing the risk of barotrauma.

Pharmacologic Interventions

Aminophylline:
Despite limited evidence of efficacy in adults, intravenous aminophylline (loading dose of 5 mg/kg over 20 minutes, followed by 0.3 -- 0.6 mg/kg/h) may be considered in rare cases of treatment-resistant asthma under specialist

supervision, particularly in patients not taking oral xanthines.

Antibiotics:
Routine antibiotic use is not recommended unless there is clear evidence of infection.

Ketamine:
Ketamine's potential in asthma management is attributed to its sympathomimetic effects, direct smooth muscle relaxation, histamine antagonism, and membrane stabilization. A randomized trial showed no significant benefit at sub-induction doses. However, in intubated patients, ketamine infusion (bolus of 1 mg/kg, followed by 1 mg/kg/h) has demonstrated improvements in gas exchange, dynamic compliance, and ventilation parameters.

Patient Disposition and Criteria for Admission

Discharge Considerations:

Patients with mild asthma can typically be discharged with a treatment plan. For moderate or severe asthma:

Post-treatment PEFR >70% predicted: Safe for discharge on appropriate therapy.

Post-treatment PEFR 40–70% predicted: Observation and extended treatment in an ED unit are necessary.

Post-treatment PEFR <40% predicted: Requires hospital admission.

Additional factors influencing discharge include:

Previous near-fatal episodes or frequent hospitalizations

Recent steroid use or sudden exacerbations

Poor adherence to treatment or suboptimal home circumstances

ICU/High-Dependency Unit Admission Criteria: Admission is warranted for:

Deteriorating PEFR

Persistent or worsening hypoxia

Hypercapnia or acidosis

Respiratory exhaustion or altered consciousness

Need for ventilatory assistance or respiratory arrest

Post-Discharge Planning

All discharged patients should receive an individualized asthma action plan outlining steps to manage potential worsening over the next 24–48 hours. Follow-up arrangements, either with a hospital team or general practitioner, should be scheduled within this timeframe. Medications upon discharge should align with prior treatment protocols.

References

1. Holgate, S.T. (2011). Pathophysiology of asthma: Insights into new therapeutic strategies. Journal of Allergy and Clinical Immunology, 128(3), 495–505.

2. Murphy, D.M., & O'Byrne, P.M. (2010). Recent developments in asthma pathophysiology. Chest, 137(6), 1417–1426.

3. Kelly, A.M. (2010). Venous blood gas analysis as a potential alternative to arterial blood gas in emergency care: A review. Emergency Medicine Australasia, 22(6), 493–498.

4. Haney, S., & Hancox, R.J. (2007). Overcoming beta-agonist tolerance through

high-dose salbutamol and ipratropium bromide: Results from two randomized controlled trials. Respiratory Research, 8, 19.

5. Rowe, B.H., Bretzlaff, J., & Bourdon, C. (2000). The role of magnesium sulfate in the treatment of acute asthma exacerbations in the emergency department. Cochrane Database of Systematic Reviews, 1, CD001490.

6. Kew, K.M., Kirtchuk, L., Michell, C.I., & Griffiths, B. (2014). Intravenous magnesium sulfate for the treatment of acute asthma in adults in the emergency department: A protocol. Cochrane Database of Systematic Reviews, 1, CD010909.

7. Bond, K.R., Horsley, C.A., & Williams, A.B. (2017). Non-invasive ventilation in status : A 16-year experience in a tertiary intensive care setting. Emergency Medicine Australasia. [epub ahead of print].

8. Parameswaran, K., Belda, J., & Rowe, B.H. (2000). Intravenous aminophylline added to beta2-agonists for acute asthma management in adults: A Cochrane review. Cochrane Database of Systematic Reviews, 4, CD002742.

9. Goyal, S., & Agrawal, A. (2013). The use of ketamine in : A comprehensive review. Indian Journal of Critical Care Medicine, 17(3), 154–161.

Chapter 4
Community-Acquired Pneumonia

Key points

1. Definition: Community-acquired pneumonia (CAP) refers to an acute lower respiratory tract infection accompanied by a new infiltrate on chest x-ray (CXR) in a patient who has not been hospitalized in the 14 days preceding the diagnosis.

2. CXR Limitations: Recent studies suggest that CXR may not be as reliable for diagnosing pneumonia, especially in elderly patients or those with comorbidities such as congestive heart failure (CCF) or chronic obstructive pulmonary disease (COPD). While computed tomography (CT) provides more detailed imaging, it remains too resource- and radiation-intensive for routine use in pneumonia diagnosis.

3. Severity Assessment: Severity scoring systems like SMART-COP and CORB are used to assess the severity of pneumonia and guide treatment decisions, including the site of care and antibiotic therapy. The Pneumonia Severity Index (PSI) and CURB-65 are useful for identifying low-risk patients who can be treated at home.

4. Causative Agents: Streptococcus pneumoniae is the most common bacterial cause of CAP. However, the proportion of cases attributed to this pathogen may have decreased due to the use of pneumococcal vaccines. Other causative organisms vary based on patient demographics, disease severity, and seasonal epidemics. Regional knowledge of local pathogens and their antibiotic resistance patterns is important for appropriate empiric antibiotic prescribing.

5. Antibiotic Therapy: The primary treatment for CAP includes beta-lactams combined with either macrolides or tetracyclines. Respiratory fluoroquinolones may also be effective but

should be used with caution due to concerns about cost, emerging resistance, and complications such as Clostridium difficile infections.

6. Guideline Use: Adherence to locally adapted, structured guidelines for managing CAP has been shown to improve patient outcomes and reduce mortality.

Introduction

Community-acquired pneumonia (CAP) presents as a spectrum of disease severity, ranging from mild and self-limiting to severe and potentially life-threatening. Many CAP cases, often without radiological confirmation, are managed in the community with oral antibiotics. In the emergency department, the primary challenge lies not in diagnosing CAP itself, but in distinguishing between serious cases that require inpatient care and those that can be managed effectively at home. While urgent and life-threatening CAP cases requiring critical interventions are uncommon, they do occur.

Chest x-ray (CXR) has long been regarded as the gold standard for pneumonia diagnosis. However, with the increased use of advanced imaging techniques and concerns about inter-rater variability in CXR interpretation, there is growing uncertainty about its reliability. This issue is exacerbated in the elderly population, who often have multiple comorbidities that can complicate CXR interpretation. Despite these concerns, CXR remains the first-line investigation for most patients due to its cost-effectiveness and relatively low radiation exposure compared to alternative imaging options. Additional tests, such as the urinary antigen test (UAT), sputum and blood cultures, inflammatory markers, and renal and liver function tests, may be useful in selected cases. A strategic approach to diagnostic testing can help reduce unnecessary healthcare costs and prevent inappropriate decisions based on misleading results.

Antibiotic management of CAP has remained relatively unchanged over the years. However, the advent of respiratory fluoroquinolones like moxifloxacin and levofloxacin has expanded treatment options. Drug-resistant pathogens, including Streptococcus pneumoniae (DRSP) and community-acquired methicillin-resistant Staphylococcus aureus (CA-MRSA), have introduced new challenges in managing CAP.

In the past two decades, comprehensive, evidence-based guidelines from organizations such as the British Thoracic Society (BTS) and the Infectious Diseases Society of America and American Thoracic Society (IDSA/ATS), as well as international groups in Australia, Japan, Sweden, Canada, and India, have been published. These guidelines emphasize the importance of a structured, evidence-based approach to managing CAP, which has been shown to improve patient outcomes. It is important that these guidelines be adapted to local conditions to optimize their effectiveness.

Epidemiology

Accurately estimating the rates of CAP is difficult due to challenges in case definition and the fact that many cases are not studied in clinical settings. International studies suggest an incidence of 5 to 11 per 1,000 individuals per year in those aged 16 to 59, and over 30 per 1,000 in those aged 75 and older. In the United Kingdom, the rate of hospitalization for CAP is less than 5 per 1,000, representing less than 50% of all CAP cases. On the other hand, CAP accounts for 8% to 10% of intensive care unit (ICU) admissions.

ICU admission rates for CAP vary widely, reflecting differences in healthcare resources and practice rather than disease severity. Studies in New Zealand report ICU admission rates of 1% to 3%, while in the United Kingdom the figure is approximately 5%, and in Australia it reaches 10%. The United States reports higher rates.

The mortality rate for community-treated CAP is thought to be very low, typically less than 1%. However, for hospitalized patients, the mortality rate is estimated at 5% to 10%, and among those requiring ICU care, mortality can be considerably higher, with variability based on ICU admission criteria. Mortality rates are also influenced by disease severity and the type of pathogen. For example, Staphylococcus aureus, gram-negative bacilli (especially Pseudomonas), Burkholderia pseudomallei, and Legionella species are associated with higher mortality rates, while pathogens like Mycoplasma and Chlamydophila species are linked to lower mortality.

In Australia, pneumonia and influenza account for approximately 2.3% of all deaths, and contribute to illness in 13.3% of cases.

Pathogenesis and Aetiology

Most cases of CAP result from the aspiration of normal flora from the upper respiratory tract. However, pathogens such as Legionella species and Mycobacterium tuberculosis may also be aspirated via aerosolized droplets. Hematogenous spread from distant infection sources, such as right-sided endocarditis, can also lead to pneumonia.

In healthy individuals, large-volume aspiration is typically prevented by intact gag and cough reflexes. However, microaspiration occurs regularly during sleep and is usually cleared by the mucociliary escalator and periodic coughing. The respiratory tract's defenses, including a layer of mucus rich in immunoglobulin A (IgA), work to prevent pathogen adhesion and activation of other immune system components. Despite these defenses, opportunistic organisms, including gram-negative rods, anaerobes, Staphylococcus aureus, and fungi, can breach these barriers and cause infection.

Identifying the exact pathogen responsible for CAP can be challenging. Studies have shown that a causative organism is identified in only around 40% of cases in hospital-based studies, with lower rates in community settings. A survey by the Centers for Disease Control (CDC) found that viral agents were responsible for 24% of hospitalized CAP cases, while bacteria were identified in only 14%.

Common Pathogens in CAP

1. Streptococcus pneumoniae
Streptococcus pneumoniae (pneumococcus) is the most commonly identified bacterial pathogen in CAP, though its prevalence has declined in recent years, likely due to widespread pneumococcal vaccination. Pneumococcus remains the predominant bacterial cause of CAP, responsible for approximately 5% of cases in some studies. The incidence of penicillin-resistant Streptococcus pneumoniae (DRSP) is rising globally. In Australia, approximately 12% to 20% of S. pneumoniae

isolates exhibit intermediate sensitivity to penicillin, though high-level resistance remains rare.

2. Mycoplasma pneumoniae

Mycoplasma pneumoniae is a common cause of CAP, particularly in younger individuals. It lacks a cell wall, making it resistant to beta-lactam antibiotics. Diagnosis is typically based on serological tests, as these organisms are difficult to culture. Mycoplasma pneumoniae accounts for 10% to 15% of CAP cases and generally causes mild, self-limiting disease, although it can lead to complications in individuals with certain pre-existing conditions.

3. Legionella species

Legionella species, which are often associated with contaminated water sources, account for a small percentage of mild and moderate CAP cases but are overrepresented in severe cases, particularly in ICU settings. Legionella infections tend to be multisystemic and are often associated with high morbidity and mortality.

4. Staphylococcus aureus

Staphylococcus aureus is a major pathogen in severe cases of CAP and is commonly associated with ICU admissions. This bacterium is known for its high resistance to penicillin and is a significant contributor to morbidity and mortality in severe pneumonia cases.

Clinical Investigations in Pneumonia Diagnosis and Management

Imaging Techniques

1. Chest X-ray (CXR)

CXR remains a fundamental tool in diagnosing pneumonia, with the presence of a new infiltrate often being key to the diagnosis. However, its reliability can be compromised, especially in elderly patients or those with underlying pulmonary diseases like chronic obstructive pulmonary disease (COPD) or congestive cardiac failure (CCF). In these populations, CXR may show inconsistent results, though it still serves as a diagnostic reference when used alongside clinical evaluation. While a normal chest examination makes pneumonia unlikely, reliance on CXR alone has limitations.

CXR can provide valuable insights into the potential etiology of pneumonia. For example:

Mycoplasma pneumonia is less likely when homogeneous lung shadowing is observed but may be suggested by accompanying lymphadenopathy.

Bacteremic streptococcal pneumonia is more probable with multilobar infiltrates or pleural effusions.

Staphylococcus aureus pneumonia may present with multilobar infiltrates, pneumatoceles, cavitation, or pneumothorax.

Klebsiella pneumonia typically affects the right upper lobe, though the connection with a bulging horizontal fissure lacks strong evidence.

Tuberculosis (TB) should be considered if an upper lobe infiltrate is seen, particularly when there is evidence of a Ghon focus or calcified nodule.

The role of repeat CXR is debated, with improvement rates varying across patients. The presence of comorbidities or more severe pneumonia may result in slower radiological improvement, particularly with pathogens like Legionella or bacteremic Streptococcus. A follow-up CXR may be considered in patients with risk factors for underlying lung cancer, especially those over 50 years of age who smoke.

2. Computed Tomography (CT)

CT scanning is increasingly used in diagnosing pneumonia, particularly when performed to assess other conditions. However, CT is not practical for routine pneumonia diagnosis due to its higher costs, radiation exposure, and time requirements.

3. Ultrasound

Lung ultrasound is a promising tool in emergency settings, showing potential as an alternative when CXR is unavailable or delayed. While its sensitivity and specificity typically reach around 85%, performance can vary depending on the clinical context. This technique is particularly useful when imaging delays occur, provided the operator is skilled.

General Pathology Testing

Full Blood Count (FBC):
FBC is routinely measured in hospitalized pneumonia patients. Anemia, thrombocytopenia,

and significant leukocytosis or leukopenia may indicate the severity of the condition. Polycythemia can suggest dehydration or chronic hypoxia. An elevated white blood cell count ($>15,000/mm^3$) often points to bacterial infections, especially Streptococcus pneumoniae, but is not a specific marker for pneumonia.

Urea and Electrolytes:
Serum urea, electrolytes, and creatinine are essential tests in managing pneumonia. Hyponatremia (Na < 130 mmol/L) and elevated urea ($\geq$ 11 mmol/L) are indicators of severe pneumonia. Acute renal impairment can complicate pneumonia, particularly in patients with pre-existing kidney disease.

Liver Function Tests:
Abnormal liver function tests are common, though they often do not directly influence management decisions. Chronic liver disease increases the risk of severe pneumonia, while hypoalbuminemia may signal worsening disease severity.

Blood Gas Testing:

Arterial blood gas (ABG) testing is routinely used in hospitalized pneumonia patients to evaluate acid-base balance and oxygenation. Some studies support the use of venous blood gasses as an alternative, which may be more practical for assessing hypercapnia. Pulse oximetry (SpO_2) is another acceptable tool for monitoring oxygen levels, though its accuracy diminishes at values below 90%.

Inflammatory Markers:

C-reactive protein (CRP) measurement is a debated practice; while it doesn't directly indicate severity, it may differentiate pneumonia from other conditions like COPD exacerbations. In outpatient settings, a negative CRP may help reduce unnecessary antibiotic use. Serum procalcitonin, D-dimer, and cortisol levels are also studied as markers of pneumonia severity, but their clinical utility remains uncertain.

Microbiological Testing

Accurately identifying the pathogen responsible for community-acquired pneumonia (CAP) is challenging, though it remains a goal in both clinical and research settings. Identifying the causative agent can inform targeted therapy and help detect outbreaks or bioterrorism events. However, pursuing a definitive diagnosis can be costly, time-consuming, and may lead to delays in treatment.

1. Sputum Collection:
Sputum samples can be collected for both microscopy and culture, although many patients cannot produce sputum, delaying antibiotic initiation. Microscopy (using Gram stain or Ziehl-Neelsen for tuberculosis) provides preliminary guidance, while sputum culture offers more detailed results, including organism identification and antibiotic sensitivity. However, sputum culture results are not available immediately, and early antibiotic therapy can reduce culture sensitivity.

Specialized culture media are required for identifying organisms like Legionella or Mycobacterium tuberculosis.

2. Blood Culture:

Blood cultures are often recommended for hospitalized pneumonia patients. However, their yield is low, with positive results occurring in only 7% of cases. Blood cultures are more beneficial when a non-pneumococcal pathogen is suspected, or in patients with severe illness or those at risk of resistant organisms. A positive blood culture result, while uncommon, is a highly specific indicator of the pathogen's role in the infection.

3. Urinary Antigen Testing (UAT):

Urinary antigen tests for Legionella and Streptococcus pneumoniae are quick and minimally impacted by prior antibiotic use. The pneumococcal UAT has high specificity (over 90%) but moderate sensitivity (50-80%). The

Legionella UAT is sensitive for L. serogroup 1 but does not detect other Legionella species or serogroups. A positive result for Legionella may suggest a more severe infection, though it should not be used to adjust initial antibiotic therapy in all cases.

4. Serology:

Serologic testing plays a limited role in emergency settings but is helpful in investigating suspected outbreaks of viral or atypical pneumonia. Paired serological tests conducted weeks apart can confirm infections like Mycoplasma or Legionella, though these tests are not practical for immediate management.

Severity Assessment

Determining the severity of CAP is crucial, as most cases are mild and self-limiting, but appropriate management is essential to prevent complications. Severe cases, often requiring hospitalization or ICU admission, demand more intensive monitoring and intervention. Factors such as age, comorbidities, and clinical signs of distress are key to assessing pneumonia severity and guiding treatment decisions.

The CURB-65 Score: Simplified and Evidence-Based Approach

The CURB-65 score is an essential tool recommended by the British Thoracic Society (BTS) for stratifying the severity of community-acquired pneumonia (CAP). This scoring system helps healthcare providers assess the risk of mortality and determine appropriate care for patients based on a score ranging from 0 to 5. A point is given for each of the following factors:

1. Confusion: New onset of confusion, as indicated by an AMTS (Abbreviated Mental Test Score) below 8 or disorientation in time, place, or person.

2. Urea: A serum urea level greater than 7 mmol/L.

3. Respiratory Rate: A respiratory rate of 30 breaths per minute or higher.

4. Blood Pressure: Systolic blood pressure below 90 mmHg or diastolic pressure $\leq$ 60 mmHg.

5. Age: Patients aged 65 years or older.

Each component of the CURB-65 score contributes to identifying the patient's overall risk of mortality and informs decisions regarding the site of care. Lower scores (0 or 1) often indicate that patients can be safely managed at home, while higher scores (2 or more) suggest the need for hospitalization and possibly more intensive care.

The CURB-65 score has been extensively validated across a wide range of patient populations in the United Kingdom and internationally. Its simplicity and ease of use have made it a reliable tool for emergency department (ED) staff and clinicians managing CAP. It performs comparably to other scoring systems, such as the Pneumonia Severity Index (PSI) and ATS (American Thoracic Society) scores, particularly in identifying low-risk patients who may be safely treated at home. However, it should be noted that while CURB-65 and PSI are effective in identifying patients for outpatient care, neither is particularly reliable in predicting the need for intensive care unit (ICU) admission or the risk of death.

The CRB-65 score, a simplified version of CURB-65 without the urea measurement, offers similar predictive power and may be used in clinical settings where urea testing is not immediately available. In particular, a CRB-65 score of 0 indicates that a patient is low-risk and can usually be managed safely in the community.

Clinical Application and Limitations

While the CURB-65 score provides valuable guidance, it is not a substitute for clinical judgment. Several factors must be considered when determining the appropriate care plan. For instance, young patients, despite potentially higher scores, may have good outcomes, while older, frail individuals with lower scores may require hospitalization even for mild pneumonia. Factors such as need for supplemental oxygen, the patient's living conditions (e.g., homelessness, unreliable social support), and the presence of comorbidities should always be considered.

In practice, patients with CURB-65 scores of 0 or 1 are typically candidates for outpatient treatment, provided that they can be adequately monitored and meet the criteria for safe home care. For patients with scores of 2 or higher, a period of supervised inpatient care is recommended to ensure proper antibiotic administration and close monitoring for deterioration.

For those requiring ICU care, scoring systems like SMART-COP or CORB may be more helpful in determining the need for critical care. However, regular re-assessment by an experienced clinician is essential to ensure that treatment decisions remain appropriate.

Treatment and Antibiotic Management

The initial treatment for CAP is almost always empiric, as the exact pathogen may not be immediately identifiable. Broad-spectrum antibiotics are selected to cover the most common and likely pathogens. For typical pneumonia caused by Streptococcus pneumoniae, beta-lactam antibiotics are commonly used. Atypical organisms like Mycoplasma pneumoniae, Legionella spp., and Chlamydia pneumoniae are typically covered with macrolides or tetracyclines.

However, emerging antibiotic resistance is a growing concern. For example, macrolide-resistant Streptococcus pneumoniae is more common in certain regions, particularly in Asia, and this impacts treatment decisions. In these cases, it may be necessary to add a beta-lactam antibiotic to ensure sufficient coverage.

The decision to escalate or change antibiotic therapy is typically based on clinical factors, including the severity of illness, the likelihood of drug-resistant pathogens, and the patient's clinical response. In cases of severe pneumonia, empiric therapy should cover a broader range of potential pathogens, including Staphylococcus aureus, Gram-negative bacilli, and Pseudomonas aeruginosa.

Management of Mild, Moderate, and Severe Pneumonia

1. Mild Pneumonia: Patients who are stable enough to be treated at home are typically given

oral antibiotics, with amoxicillin often the preferred first-line treatment. In some cases, additional coverage for atypical pathogens with a macrolide may be appropriate, especially during periods of Mycoplasma pneumoniae outbreaks.

2. Moderate Pneumonia: Hospitalized patients typically receive intravenous beta-lactam antibiotics combined with a tetracycline like doxycycline or a third-generation cephalosporin. In cases where penicillin allergies are suspected, alternative antibiotics are used.

3. Severe Pneumonia: In severe cases, empiric therapy must be broad to cover potential pathogens such as S. aureus, Legionella spp., and Gram-negative organisms. If necessary, therapy is adjusted based on microbiological findings, with the goal of ensuring adequate coverage while avoiding overuse of broad-spectrum antibiotics.

Conclusion

The CURB-65 score provides a straightforward, evidence-based method for guiding treatment decisions in CAP. It is particularly useful for determining whether a patient can be safely treated at home or should be admitted to the hospital. While it is a valuable tool, the score should always be used in conjunction with clinical judgment and other considerations, such as patient comorbidities, social circumstances, and oxygenation status. Antibiotic management must balance the need for broad coverage with the risks of overuse, particularly in the face of rising antibiotic resistance. By applying these principles, clinicians can optimize patient care and reduce the burden of pneumonia-related morbidity and mortality.

References

1. Lim WS, Baudouin SV, George RC, et al. The BTS guidelines for managing

community-acquired pneumonia in adults: 2009 update. Thorax. 2009; Suppl 3: iii1-55.

2. Buising KL, Thursky KA, Black JF. Identifying severe community-acquired pneumonia in the emergency department: a clinical prediction tool. Emerg Med Australas. 2007;19(5):418–426.

3. Charles PG, Whitby M, Fuller AJ, et al. The etiology of community-acquired pneumonia in Australia: optimal therapy with penicillin plus doxycycline or a macrolide. Clin Infect Dis. 2008;46(10):1513–1521.

4. Charles PG, Wolfe R, Whitby M, et al. SMART-COP: a predictive tool for assessing the need for intensive respiratory or vasopressor support in community-acquired pneumonia. Clin Infect Dis. 2008;47(3):375–384.

5. Community Acquired Pneumonia. In: eTG Complete (CD-ROM). Melbourne: Therapeutic Guidelines Ltd; 2017 (updated November 2014).

6. Elliott JH, Anstey NM, Jacups SP, et al. Community-acquired pneumonia in northern Australia: low mortality in a tropical region using locally developed treatment guidelines. Int J Infect Dis. 2005;9(1):15–20.

7. Fine MJ, Auble TE, Yealy DM, et al. A prediction rule for identifying low-risk patients with community-acquired pneumonia. N Engl J Med. 1997;336(4):243–250.

8. Jain S, Self WH, Wunderink RG, Fakhran S, et al. Hospitalized adults with community-acquired pneumonia in the U.S. N Engl J Med. 2015;373:415–427.

9. Kennedy M, Bates DW, Wright SB, et al. Impact of emergency department blood cultures on pneumonia treatment practices. Ann Emerg Med. 2005;46(5):393–400.

10. Mandell LA, Wunderink RG, Anzueto A, et al. Infectious Diseases Society of

America/American Thoracic Society consensus guidelines for managing community-acquired pneumonia in adults. Clin Infect Dis. 2007;44(suppl 2):S27–S72.

11. Shefet D, Robenstone, Paul M, Leibovici L. Empiric antibiotic coverage of atypical pathogens for hospitalized adults with community-acquired pneumonia. Cochrane Database Syst Rev. 2005;(2):CD00

Chapter 5
Influenza and Emerging Respiratory Infections

Key points

1. Influenza is contagious even before symptoms develop.

2. The most common complications of influenza are pneumonia and exacerbations of pre-existing chronic conditions.

3. Clinical signs have low sensitivity and specificity, making polymerase chain reaction (PCR) testing crucial for accurate diagnosis.

4. The use of antiviral therapy remains debated, but it is beneficial in treating certain patient populations.

5. Nosocomial transmission poses a significant risk to both patient and staff safety, as well as

emergency department (ED) operations. The early identification and proper use of personal protective equipment (PPE) at triage are essential for safeguarding both patients and healthcare workers.

6. Vaccination against influenza for high-risk groups and healthcare personnel is the most effective preventive measure.

7. Emergency preparedness for both seasonal and pandemic influenza should be viewed as an ongoing process, with response efforts escalating based on patient volume, staff absenteeism, and patient severity.

Introduction

Influenza is an infectious respiratory disease caused by an RNA virus from the Orthomyxoviridae family. It is a highly contagious condition that typically affects between 5% and 10% of adults and 20% to 30%

of children annually. The mortality rate varies from 1.4 to 16.7 deaths per 100,000 people. Seasonal influenza epidemics result in 3 to 5 million severe cases and 290,000 to 650,000 deaths worldwide every year. The highest mortality rates occur in elderly individuals, infants, and immunocompromised patients, with notable morbidity and loss of productivity seen due to worker absenteeism and school closures. General practice clinics, emergency departments, and hospitals often experience significant strain during peak influenza seasons. Influenza pandemics, caused by mutations that lead to the emergence of new virus strains, can disrupt both the healthcare sector and the global economy.

Microbiological Classification

Influenza viruses are classified into three main types: A, B, and C, based on their core proteins. Types A and B are responsible for seasonal epidemics, while type C causes rare respiratory illnesses and does not typically lead to epidemics. Influenza A is the most virulent and tends to cause the most severe disease. The influenza A virus is further subdivided into subtypes based on two surface proteins: haemagglutinin (H) and neuraminidase (N). There are 18 different subtypes of haemagglutinin and 11 subtypes of neuraminidase. Haemagglutinin facilitates viral attachment to host cell receptors, and neuraminidase plays a key role in viral release from infected cells, allowing the virus to spread. Both proteins are targets for antiviral drugs. Influenza B viruses are not categorized into subtypes but are divided into lineages and strains, including the B/Yamagata and B/Victoria lineages. Influenza viruses are named based on their antigenic type, host origin, geographical origin, strain number, and the year of isolation. For example, type A viruses are further classified by their H and N subtypes, such as H1N1 or H5N1.

Epidemiology

Antigenic drift refers to small changes in the antigenicity of haemagglutinin or neuraminidase, typically caused by point mutations. These mutations help the virus evade immune detection and are responsible for most seasonal influenza epidemics. In contrast, antigenic shift is a more significant change in the antigenicity of the virus, resulting from genetic reassortment between different influenza A subtypes during co-infection of a single host. This can also occur through reassortment between animal and human influenza strains, creating novel antigens that the human immune system does not recognize. This process can potentially lead to a lethal pandemic. Notable influenza pandemics include the 1918 Spanish flu (H1N1), which caused an estimated 30 to 50 million deaths, as well as the 1957 Asian flu (H2N2), the 1968 Hong Kong flu (H3N2), and the 2009 swine flu (H1N1).

Avian and Other Zoonotic Influenzas

The binding specificity of haemagglutinin restricts the transmission of zoonotic influenza strains, such as avian influenza (H5N1, H7N9) and swine flu (H1N1, H3N2). Transmission to humans requires direct or indirect contact with infected animals, which can occur in wet markets or during the slaughtering and preparation of animals for food. Person-to-person transmission typically requires close contact, such as during caregiving or medical procedures that generate airborne respiratory droplets. Zoonotic influenza viruses cannot be transmitted through properly cooked food. Since 1997, the H5N1 avian influenza virus has spread from Asia to Europe and Africa, becoming endemic in many poultry populations. In 2013, H7N9 infections emerged in China, with cases later reported in other parts of Asia. Despite the high human mortality associated with these viruses, they are not yet capable of sustained human-to-human transmission. However, they remain a significant pandemic threat due to their high mortality rate and global spread in animal populations.

Incubation Period and Infectivity

Influenza's incubation period is typically around 2 days, though it can range from 1 to 4 days. Transmission primarily occurs through respiratory droplets from sneezing and coughing, but can also happen via direct or indirect contact with contaminated surfaces. Healthcare workers are at elevated risk of contracting influenza, which can lead to hospital-associated infections, especially among vulnerable patients. An infected individual is contagious from the day before symptoms appear until 5 to 7 days after symptom onset, with children and immunocompromised individuals potentially remaining contagious for up to 3 weeks. The severity of the illness correlates with the amount of virus shed, which is influenced by fever intensity. Previous influenza vaccination or prior infections with similar strains can offer partial protection. Influenza viruses thrive in cold, low-humidity conditions, which is why seasonal epidemics primarily occur in winter. The virus can survive for 24 to 48 hours on hard, non-porous surfaces, 8 to 12 hours on soft surfaces like cloth or paper, and up to 5 minutes on hands. Disinfectants effectively inactivate the virus.

Clinical Features

The hallmark of uncomplicated influenza is the sudden onset of symptoms such as fever, chills, muscle aches, headaches, and fatigue, followed by respiratory symptoms like sore throat and a dry cough. Nasal congestion is possible but less common. Gastrointestinal symptoms, including nausea, vomiting, and diarrhea, are more frequent in children, who may also develop otitis media. Examination typically reveals fever (37.8°C–40.0°C), rapid heart rate, and a reddened throat without exudate. While influenza affects individuals across all age groups, its severity can range from mild to life-threatening, with respiratory failure and death being potential outcomes. People with partial immunity due to prior infections or vaccinations tend to experience milder illness. Symptoms generally resolve within 5 to 7 days, though fatigue and cough may persist for up to 2 weeks. High-risk groups, including the elderly, young children, pregnant women, and those with chronic or immunocompromising conditions, are more likely to experience complications, hospitalization, or death.

Complications

Influenza can worsen existing medical conditions, such as congestive heart failure, asthma, and chronic obstructive pulmonary disease (COPD). Pneumonia is the most common and severe complication, which can be viral, bacterial, or a mix of both. Secondary bacterial pneumonia is marked by a return of fever and worsening respiratory symptoms after an initial improvement, often accompanied by purulent sputum. Common causative bacteria include Streptococcus pneumoniae, Staphylococcus aureus, and Haemophilus influenzae. Staphylococcal pneumonia, particularly from methicillin-resistant strains, is associated with a high mortality rate. Primary viral pneumonia, while less common, is more severe and can progress to acute respiratory distress syndrome (ARDS) and organ failure. Elderly individuals, pregnant women, and those with cardiovascular disease are most at risk for primary viral pneumonia. Avian influenza (H5N1) often leads to primary viral pneumonia, with ARDS and respiratory failure occurring in 60% of confirmed cases. Other non-respiratory complications can include myositis, rhabdomyolysis, myocarditis, pericarditis, encephalitis, aseptic meningitis, transverse myelitis, and Guillain-Barré syndrome. syndrome may also develop in children taking aspirin for influenza.

Differential Diagnosis

Influenza shares symptoms with many other respiratory infections, so careful differentiation is essential, particularly from bacterial sepsis, other viral infections, and emerging respiratory diseases like SARS and MERS. The diagnosis of influenza is more likely when the onset is abrupt, accompanied by high fever and constitutional symptoms such as headache, muscle pain, joint pain, or lethargy. Case definitions of influenza typically include fever (>38.5°C), at least one constitutional symptom, and one respiratory symptom (cough or sore throat). The sensitivity and specificity of these definitions can vary depending on the patient group and time of year, with lower sensitivity observed in elderly and immunocompromised individuals who may not exhibit typical symptoms. Microbiological testing is required to definitively diagnose influenza.

Clinical Investigations

Blood tests in influenza patients typically show a normal white blood cell count, with lymphopenia being a common feature. A high white blood cell count (greater than 15,000/μL) may suggest pneumonia, either viral or bacterial, while moderately elevated C-reactive protein (CRP) levels (<100) can be indicative of infection, though it is more useful when combined with other clinical signs.

Imaging studies, such as chest X-rays, are recommended for patients with severe symptoms or pulmonary concerns. Primary viral pneumonia typically presents as diffuse reticular or reticulonodular infiltrates, while bacterial pneumonia often shows focal consolidation. Multiple cavities on imaging are indicative of S. aureus infection.

Influenza Preparedness in Healthcare Settings

Hospitals and emergency departments (EDs) must establish and regularly practice their own guidelines for managing influenza. Both seasonal and pandemic influenza management should be viewed as an ongoing process, with escalation of response based on factors such as patient volume, the severity of illness, and staff absenteeism due to illness.

At a fundamental level, the guidelines should emphasize essential infection control measures, such as hand hygiene, aseptic techniques, adherence to standard precautions and transmission-based precautions, and appropriate use of personal protective equipment (PPE). Encouraging high vaccination rates among healthcare staff against influenza and other vaccine-preventable diseases is critical.

Screening and Triage

Screening for influenza-like illnesses (ILIs) should be conducted during the triage process. The screening methods will depend on the ED's capacity, but they should include inquiries about symptoms such as fever, with or without a cough. Additionally, the presence of risk factors such as immunosuppression, contact with sick individuals, and recent international travel should be assessed. The distribution of case definitions for influenza or ILI to healthcare staff can help guide clinical management. Research indicates that the combination of fever and cough has a high sensitivity (77%), though its specificity is lower (33%).

Patients identified as having an ILI should be provided with a surgical mask, and directed to hand hygiene stations in the waiting room. If possible, they should be seated at least 1 meter away from other patients. Those requiring triage in a cubicle should be placed in a single room with appropriate signage indicating the need for droplet isolation precautions. Healthcare workers should use surgical masks and gloves when caring for these patients.

Managing Unsafe Practices and Aerosolization

Certain practices may increase the risk of aerosolizing the virus, such as nebulizing medications. When nebulization is necessary, additional precautions should be taken to reduce the risk of airborne transmission. These precautions should include the use of negative pressure rooms, along with full PPE, including impervious gowns, N95 masks, face shields, and gloves. In the absence of negative pressure rooms, a regular room with the door closed and appropriate PPE should be used. A single room used for nebulization should not be reused by other patients for at least 1 hour to allow viral particles to clear from the air.

Role of Flu Clinics in Preparedness

Hospital influenza preparedness guidelines should also include the establishment of flu clinics to support continuity of care during influenza outbreaks. Decisions about setting up these clinics should involve discussions between adjacent healthcare facilities, medical administration, emergency departments, and inpatient services. The threshold for establishing flu clinics will depend on the increase in ED visits, patient severity, and staffing capacity. The guidelines should include specifics on the location, staffing, operating hours, and funding of flu clinics, and should also address the criteria for decommissioning them.

PPE and Antiviral Medication Supply

Guidelines should specify the quantities of PPE and antiviral drugs, including neuraminidase inhibitors, that are available. State health departments will determine whether antivirals should be given to frontline healthcare workers, such as ED staff. During the 2009 H1N1 pandemic, neuraminidase inhibitors were not prescribed to responders, and emphasis was placed on strict infection control practices and appropriate use of PPE.

Ethical Considerations

Ethical concerns in influenza preparedness should focus on advance care planning. Emergency department staff should explore both value-based and treatment-based directives with patients, when appropriate. Hospitals involved in nursing home care should provide appropriate options for care outside the acute setting, especially for vulnerable populations.

Emerging Respiratory Infections (ERIs)

Emerging Respiratory Infections are defined as novel or evolving infections, including changes in drug resistance, virulence, and transmission patterns. This category includes MERS-CoV, pandemic influenza, and other potential threats. Activation of seasonal influenza plans is the most effective strategy to protect both staff and patients during the emergence of an ERI. ED staff are often among the first healthcare workers to be exposed to such infections, highlighting the importance of strong infection control practices and the use of PPE in all patient interactions.

Controversies in Influenza Management

The issue of mandatory influenza vaccination for healthcare workers, including opt-out provisions.

The clinical efficacy and cost-effectiveness of neuraminidase inhibitors.

The use of Extracorporeal Membrane Oxygenation (ECMO) in severe cases of influenza.

References

1. World Health Organization (WHO). Influenza vaccine. Available at: http://www.who.int/biologicals/vaccines/influenza/en/. Accessed January 26, 2018.

2. Centers for Disease Control and Prevention (CDC). Estimates of deaths associated with seasonal influenza—United States, 1976–2007. MMWR. 2010;59(33):1057–1062.

3. World Health Organization (WHO). Influenza (seasonal) fact sheet updated January 2018. Available at: http://www.who.int/mediacentre/factsheets/fs211/en/. Accessed January 26, 2018.

4. World Health Organization (WHO). Influenza (avian and other zoonotic) updated January 2018. Available at: http://www.who.int/mediacentre/factsheets/avian_influenza/en/. Accessed January 26, 2018.

5. Hirve S, Chadha M, Lele P, et al. Performance of case definitions used for influenza surveillance among hospitalized patients in a rural area of India. WHO Bulletin. Available at: http://www.who.int/bulletin/volumes/90/11/12-108837/en/. Accessed January 26, 2018.

6. Ebell MH. WHO downgrades status of oseltamivir. BMJ. 2017;358:j3266. Available at: http://www.bmj.com/content/358/bmj.j3266. Accessed January 26, 2018.

7. Sukhal S, Sethi J, Ganesh M, et al. Extracorporeal membrane oxygenation in severe influenza infection with respiratory failure: A systematic review and meta-analysis. Ann Card Anaesth. 2017;20(1):14–21. Available at:

https://doi.org/10.4103/0971-9784.197820.
Accessed January 15, 2018.

8. Immunise Australia Program. Influenza B: a B/Brisbane/60/2008-like virus, B: a B/Phuket/3073/2013-like virus, Influenza A (H1N1): an A/Michigan/45/2015 (H1N1) 09-like virus, A (H3N2): an A/Hong Kong/4801/2014 (H3N2) like virus. Available at:
http://www.immunise.health.gov.au/internet/im munise/publishing.nsf/Content/ATAGI-advice-in fluenza-vaccines-providers. Accessed January 26, 2018.

9. Pandemic Influenza Health.vic. Available at: http://www2.health.vic.gov.au/emergencies/emer gency-type/infectio.

10. World Health Organization (WHO). Influenza vaccine. Available at: http://www.who.int/biologicals/vaccines/influen za/en/. Accessed January 26, 2018.

11. Centers for Disease Control and Prevention (CDC). Estimates of deaths associated with seasonal influenza—United States, 1976–2007. MMWR. 2010;59(33):1057–1062.

12. World Health Organization (WHO). Influenza (seasonal) fact sheet updated January 2018. Available at: http://www.who.int/mediacentre/factsheets/fs211/en/. Accessed January 26, 2018.

13. World Health Organization (WHO). Influenza (avian and other zoonotic) updated January 2018. Available at: http://www.who.int/mediacentre/factsheets/avian_influenza/en/. Accessed January 26, 2018.

14. Hirve S, Chadha M, Lele P, et al. Performance of case definitions used for influenza surveillance among hospitalized patients in a rural area of India. WHO Bulletin. Available at: http://www.who.int/bulletin/volumes/90/11/12-108837/en/. Accessed January 26, 2018.

15. Ebell MH. WHO downgrades status of oseltamivir. BMJ. 2017;358:j3266. Available at: http://www.bmj.com/content/358/bmj.j3266. Accessed January 26, 2018.

16. Sukhal S, Sethi J, Ganesh M, et al. Extracorporeal membrane oxygenation in severe influenza infection with respiratory failure: A systematic review and meta-analysis. Ann Card Anaesth. 2017;20(1):14–21. Available at: https://doi.org/10.4103/0971-9784.197820. Accessed January 15, 2018.

17. Immunise Australia Program. Influenza B: a B/Brisbane/60/2008-like virus, B: a B/Phuket/3073/2013-like virus, Influenza A (H1N1): an A/Michigan/45/2015 (H1N1) 09-like virus, A (H3N2): an A/Hong Kong/4801/2014 (H3N2) like virus. Available at: http://www.immunise.health.gov.au/internet/im munise/publishing.nsf/Content/ATAGI-advice-in

fluenza-vaccines-providers. Accessed January 26, 2018.

18. Pandemic Influenza Health.vic. Available at: http://www2.health.vic.gov.au/emergencies/emergency-type/infectio.

Chapter 6
Chronic obstructive pulmonary disease

Key Points:

1. Chronic obstructive pulmonary disease (COPD) is a condition marked by irreversible airflow limitation.

2. While infections are the primary cause of COPD exacerbations, other potential triggers must also be considered and ruled out.

3. It is essential to regulate the oxygen flow rate to maintain an arterial oxygen saturation between 88% and 92%, balancing the correction of hypoxia with the avoidance of hyperoxic hypercapnia.

4. The use of non-invasive ventilation in cases of acute respiratory failure has been shown to decrease mortality rates, reduce the need for

intubation, and improve overall treatment outcomes.

5. For managing acute exacerbations of COPD, bronchodilators and systemic steroids are commonly recommended.

6. COPD management requires careful monitoring and therapeutic interventions to mitigate acute exacerbations and long-term progression of the disease.

Introduction

Chronic obstructive pulmonary disease (COPD) is a prevalent global health issue, contributing significantly to chronic morbidity and mortality. COPD is marked by persistent airflow limitation that is typically progressive and not fully reversible. It is commonly linked to an abnormal inflammatory response of the lungs to harmful particles or gasses. Acute exacerbations of COPD are complex events, resulting from a combination of factors involving the host, respiratory viruses, bacteria, and environmental pollutants. These exacerbations are clinically characterized by a sudden worsening of symptoms such as increased dyspnoea, cough, or sputum production, which exceed normal fluctuations and may necessitate changes in treatment. COPD is a chronic systemic disorder with diverse extrapulmonary effects and may lead to life-threatening respiratory failure during acute exacerbations.

Aetiology, Genetics, Pathogenesis, and Pathology

Cigarette smoking is the primary cause of COPD, though genetic factors like α1-antitrypsin deficiency, exposure to occupational hazards, and environmental pollution can also contribute. Interestingly, only about 30% of smokers develop significant COPD. The airflow limitation in COPD arises from a combination of mucus hypersecretion, destruction of alveolar attachments, and inflammation and fibrosis in the airways. Over time, COPD leads to worsening dyspnoea and reduced exercise capacity, and it is frequently associated with acute exacerbations, often triggered by infections. Chronic complications include pulmonary hypertension, cor pulmonale, secondary polycythaemia, bullous lung disease, osteoporosis, weight loss, and a deteriorating quality of life. Patients with COPD also have a high incidence of comorbid bronchiectasis, which worsens prognosis. These patients typically have a long history of smoking, produce more sputum, and experience more frequent exacerbations, often requiring broader antibiotic therapy due to bacterial colonization, including Pseudomonas aeruginosa.

Epidemiology
According to projections from the Global Burden of Disease Study, COPD is expected to become the fifth leading cause of disability-adjusted life years lost by 2020. In Australia, COPD affects approximately 7.5% of individuals aged 40 or older, ranking as the sixth leading cause of death in both men and women.

In New Zealand, COPD ranks as the fifth leading cause of death.

Clinical Features

History

COPD typically progresses slowly, with patients experiencing gradual deterioration in respiratory function. Most emergency department (ED) visits are due to acute exacerbations. As the disease advances, the frequency of exacerbations increases, so understanding a patient's baseline condition is crucial. Key questions to ask include:

Diagnosis: Has the patient been diagnosed with COPD, and when were symptoms first observed? Are pulmonary function tests available? Is the patient a current or former smoker, and how many pack-years? Are there any additional risk factors such as family history or $\alpha 1$-antitrypsin deficiency?

Severity: What medications is the patient using, and what is their exercise tolerance? Have they been hospitalized recently? What is their BMI, and have they experienced any weight loss?

Acute Exacerbation: What symptoms are present (e.g., fever, cough, sputum color/amount)? Is the patient able to perform basic activities (e.g., walking, eating, sleeping)? Are there any high-risk comorbidities, such as ischemic heart disease or diabetes?

Examination

COPD exacerbations can be life-threatening and require immediate airway management. Severe respiratory distress may manifest as tachypnoea, use of accessory muscles (e.g., pursed-lip breathing), altered consciousness, and cyanosis. After addressing critical issues, further examination focuses on both acute and chronic COPD features. Chronic signs can include a barrel chest, thin appearance, or signs of cor pulmonale (e.g., edema). Exacerbations may also be triggered by infections, sputum retention, or environmental factors. Important differential diagnoses include decompensated heart failure, acute coronary syndrome, and pulmonary embolism.

Classification and Stepwise Management of COPD
COPD severity is classified into three stages:

Mild: Patients may experience breathlessness only with moderate exertion and have minimal impact on daily activities. Lung function is between 60-80% of predicted FEV1, and treatment includes short-acting bronchodilators. Smoking cessation and vaccinations (pneumococcal and influenza) are key components of care.

Moderate: Patients have breathlessness with minimal exertion, some cough and sputum production, and increased exacerbations requiring steroids and antibiotics. Lung function is between 40-59% of predicted FEV1, and management includes long-acting bronchodilators and inhaled steroids, along with nutritional assessment and management of comorbidities.

Severe: Patients experience breathlessness even with minimal exertion and have significant limitations in daily activities. Lung function is usually less than 40% of predicted FEV1, and management includes home oxygen therapy and possible bronchoscopy. Advanced care planning and referrals for palliative care should be considered.

Clinical Investigations
Several investigations may be used in the assessment of an ED patient with COPD:

Bedside Tests: Pulse oximetry is crucial for assessing oxygenation, while a chest x-ray can provide insights into coexisting conditions such as pneumonia or pneumothorax.

Spirometry: Essential for diagnosing COPD, spirometry typically shows FEV1 less than 80% of predicted and an FEV1/FVC ratio below 0.7.

Electrocardiography (ECG): ECG may reveal signs of atrial fibrillation or evidence of right ventricular hypertrophy.

Venous Blood Gases (VBGs): These can provide important information on the patient's metabolic status, respiratory failure, and shock. Venous pCO2 levels can also help predict arterial hypercarbia.

Arterial Blood Gases (ABGs): These provide more precise information about oxygenation and hypercarbia, guiding therapeutic decisions, especially in acute settings.

Treatment of Acute Exacerbation of COPD in the Emergency Department

Objective: The primary goals for managing patients with COPD exacerbations in the emergency department (ED) are to confirm the diagnosis, assess disease severity, and optimize function. This includes the use of long-acting bronchodilators for symptom relief in moderate to severe cases, and inhaled glucocorticoids for those with severe disease and frequent exacerbations. Additionally, management strategies focus on preventing further deterioration, developing a self-management plan, and treating exacerbations.

The treatment approach varies based on the severity of the condition, with the understanding that decisions made for critically ill patients are primarily clinical, requiring no additional diagnostic tests to determine the need for immediate intubation.

Oxygen Therapy

Oxygen therapy aims to correct severe hypoxemia. For most COPD patients, oxygen therapy typically does not cause significant carbon dioxide retention. Hypercarbia in these patients arises from a combination of factors, including changes in pulmonary blood flow and ventilation/perfusion mismatch, rather than solely hypoventilation due to loss of hypoxic drive. Oxygen administration should be controlled to maintain SpO2 levels between 88% and 92% (corresponding to an arterial oxygen tension of 60-70 mmHg). Higher levels of oxygen (>93%-95%) may increase the risk of morbidity and mortality in patients with hypercapnic respiratory failure. Oxygen can initially be delivered via nasal prongs (0.5 to 2 L/min), with escalation to masks or reservoir masks if necessary. If hypoxia persists (SpO2 <85%), further investigation for complications, such as pneumonia, pulmonary edema, pulmonary embolism, or pneumothorax, should be conducted, and ventilatory support considered.

Non-Invasive Ventilation (NIV)

NIV, utilizing continuous positive airway pressure (CPAP) or bi-level positive airway pressure (BiPAP), is the first-line treatment for acute respiratory failure in COPD. Despite its proven benefits, NIV is underused in ED settings. Studies have shown that NIV reduces mortality rates, the need for intubation, hospital length of stay, and complication rates. It significantly improves oxygenation, acidosis, and respiratory rate within one hour of initiation. Clinical guidelines suggest NIV should be applied early in respiratory failure, before severe acidosis develops.

NIV helps reduce the work of breathing by counteracting intrinsic positive end-expiratory pressure (PEEPi), which often develops during exacerbations. CPAP and BiPAP help relieve dyspnoea, decrease respiratory fatigue, and improve gas exchange.

Indications for NIV: Moderate to severe dyspnoea, use of accessory muscles, paradoxical abdominal motion, moderate to severe acidosis and/or hypercapnia (PaCO2 >45 mmHg), and respiratory rate >25 breaths/min. Contraindications: Respiratory arrest, profound hypotension, inability to maintain an airway, uncooperative patients, vomiting, excess secretions, facial trauma, recent facial or gastro-esophageal surgery.

Approximately 85% of patients with acute respiratory failure will respond to NIV, but predicting which patients will benefit is challenging. After a successful initial response to NIV, about 20% of COPD patients will experience a second episode of respiratory failure within 48 hours.

Invasive Ventilation

Mechanical ventilation via endotracheal intubation is indicated if NIV fails or if the patient has indications for intubation from the onset, such as respiratory arrest or an unprotected airway. The goal is to prevent excessive work of breathing while maintaining enough effort to prevent respiratory muscle atrophy. Positive pressure ventilation carries risks, including barotrauma and the production of PEEPi. Ventilation strategies typically involve using tidal volumes of 5-7 mL/kg, a reduced respiratory rate, and a 1:3 inspiratory:expiratory ratio. Most patients also require intravenous fluids to counteract the effects of positive pressure ventilation on venous return and cardiac output. The mortality rate for patients requiring mechanical ventilation ranges from 17% to 30%.

When considering intubation, it is essential to weigh the patient's overall prognosis, functional baseline, and the likelihood of a successful recovery.

Bronchodilators

Bronchodilators are essential for managing acute exacerbations of COPD, as they may improve airflow obstruction, which has a reversible component. These are typically delivered via nebulizer, though metered-dose inhalers with a spacer can also be effective. Combination therapies of β2-agonists and anticholinergics are commonly used.

β2-Agonists: Salbutamol is frequently used as a first-line β2-agonist in Australia, typically given at a dose of 5 mg via nebulizer, repeated as needed. The equivalent dose via metered-dose inhaler is 8-12 puffs (100 μg each). In severe exacerbations, nebulized salbutamol may be continuously administered, or intravenous salbutamol may be required, although evidence supporting this route is limited. Common side effects include tachycardia, tremors, and reduced potassium levels.

Long-Acting β2-Agonists: Agents such as salmeterol and formoterol provide bronchodilation lasting at least 12 hours and are typically used twice daily. Although they improve lung function and reduce acute exacerbations in stable COPD, their role during acute exacerbations remains uncertain.

Anticholinergic Agents: Short-acting anticholinergics like ipratropium bromide (500 μg nebulizer every 4 to 6 hours) are frequently used, though they have a longer duration of action than short-acting β2-agonists and a lower adverse effect profile. Tiotropium, a long-acting anticholinergic, is more suitable for stable COPD but is not typically used for acute exacerbations.

Corticosteroids

Systemic corticosteroids play a critical role in reducing the severity of acute exacerbations by accelerating recovery, shortening hospital stays, and preventing relapses. Prednisolone is commonly used, with a recommended dose of 30-50 mg per day for 5 days. Oral corticosteroids are as effective as intravenous forms unless the patient cannot tolerate oral intake. Short-term corticosteroid use has a relatively low risk of adverse effects, although long-term use carries significant risks, including suppression of the hypothalamic-pituitary-adrenal axis.

Antibiotics

In approximately 50% of COPD exacerbations, bacterial infections are involved. Antibiotics are especially beneficial for patients with increased dyspnoea, sputum purulence, and volume. More severe exacerbations are more likely to benefit from antibiotics. Common pathogens include H. influenzae, S. pneumoniae, and M. . Antibiotic choices depend on local sensitivities and may include β-lactamase-resistant drugs such as ampicillin with clavulanic acid or doxycycline. In severe cases, intravenous antibiotics may be necessary.

Additional Therapies

Fluid and Nutrition Management: Monitoring fluid balance and ensuring adequate nutrition are vital components of treatment.

Correction of Electrolyte Abnormalities: It is crucial to correct any electrolyte imbalances, especially in patients with severe exacerbations.

By addressing these aspects of care in the ED, healthcare providers can improve outcomes for patients experiencing an acute exacerbation of COPD.

References

1. Vogelmeier, C. F., Criner, G. J., Martinez, F. J., et al. (2017). Global strategy for the diagnosis, management, and prevention of chronic obstructive lung disease: 2017 report – GOLD executive summary. Respirology, 22(3), 575–601.

2. Kohansal, R., Martinez-Camblor, P., Agustí, A., et al. (2009). The natural history of chronic airflow obstruction revisited: An analysis of the Framingham offspring cohort. American Journal

of Respiratory and Critical Care Medicine, 180(1), 3–10.

3. Toelle, B. G., Xuan, W., Bird, T. E., et al. (2013). Respiratory symptoms and illness in older Australians: The Burden of Obstructive Lung Disease (BOLD) study. Medical Journal of Australia, 198(3), 144–148.

4. Broekhuizen, B. D. L., Sachs, A. P. E., Oostvogels, R., et al. (2009). The diagnostic value of history and physical examination for chronic obstructive pulmonary disease in suspected or known cases: A systematic review. Family Practice, 26(4), 260–268.

5. Yang, I. A., Brown, J. L., George, J., et al. (2017). COPD-X Australian and New Zealand guidelines for the diagnosis and management of chronic obstructive pulmonary disease: 2017 update. Medical Journal of Australia, 207(10), 436–442.

6. Lim, B. L., & Kelly, A. M. (2010). A meta-analysis on the utility of peripheral venous blood gas analyses in exacerbations of chronic obstructive pulmonary disease in the emergency department. European Journal of Emergency Medicine, 17(5), 246–248.

7. Khialani, B., Sivakumaran, P., Keijzers, G., & Sriram, K. B. (2014). Emergency department management of acute exacerbations of chronic obstructive pulmonary disease and factors associated with hospitalization. Journal of Research in Medical Sciences, 19(4), 297–303.

Chapter 7
Pneumothorax

Key Points:

1. Pneumothorax can occur spontaneously, due to trauma, or as a result of medical interventions. Spontaneous pneumothorax is commonly classified into primary and secondary types, with the latter being associated with pre-existing lung diseases. However, this classification is increasingly being questioned, as there is growing evidence of underlying lung abnormalities even in individuals initially diagnosed with primary spontaneous pneumothorax.

2. Clinical symptoms alone are not reliable indicators of the size of the pneumothorax.

3. A chest X-ray is the preferred diagnostic method for pneumothorax.

4. Treatment options for pneumothorax include observation, aspiration, thoracostomy, and, depending on the case, either primary or delayed surgery. However, the available evidence to guide treatment decisions is limited.

5. Tension pneumothorax is a rare complication, particularly following a spontaneous pneumothorax. It is a medical emergency that requires immediate intervention. Diagnosis is primarily clinical rather than relying on radiological findings.

6. Smoking cessation is strongly recommended for all patients, as it significantly reduces the risk of recurrent pneumothorax.

Introduction

Pneumothorax refers to the accumulation of free air within the intrapleural space. This condition can arise spontaneously, following trauma, or as a result of medical interventions (iatrogenic causes).

Among the different types, spontaneous pneumothorax is the most prevalent, with an annual incidence of 18–28 cases per 100,000 men and 1.2–6 cases per 100,000 women. Notably, many affected individuals delay seeking medical attention, as evidenced by a study reporting that 46% of patients presented after more than two days despite experiencing symptoms.

Etiology, Pathophysiology, and Contributing Factors

Historically, spontaneous pneumothorax has been categorized into two primary types:

1. Primary Spontaneous Pneumothorax (PSP): Occurring in individuals without known lung disease.

2. Secondary Spontaneous Pneumothorax (SSP): Arising in patients with pre-existing lung conditions.

However, evolving research has challenged this binary classification. Imaging frequently identifies lung abnormalities, such as subpleural blebs, bullae, or emphysematous changes, even in PSP cases. Current perspectives suggest a continuum between PSP and SSP rather than strict delineation.

Risk Factors

PSP: More prevalent in tall, thin males aged 20–40 years. Smoking is the most significant risk factor, but there is no clear link with physical exertion.

SSP: Common in individuals aged 60–65 years and often linked to underlying conditions like chronic obstructive pulmonary disease (COPD), asthma, infections (e.g., tuberculosis, Pneumocystis jirovecii), and cystic fibrosis. Other associations include malignancies, thoracic endometriosis, and substance use (e.g., cocaine, marijuana, nitrous oxide).

Genetic Disorders: Conditions such as Marfan syndrome, Birt-Hogg-Dubé syndrome, α1-antitrypsin deficiency, and folliculin gene mutations increase susceptibility.

Iatrogenic Causes: Medical procedures like central line insertion, lung biopsy, and bronchoscopy may inadvertently introduce air into the pleural space.

Trauma: Commonly results from rib fractures, penetrating chest injuries, or barotrauma during mechanical ventilation.

Pathogenesis and Complications

In most spontaneous pneumothorax cases, air leakage resolves naturally. However, persistent air leaks can lead to a ball-valve effect, causing tension pneumothorax—a critical condition characterized by the displacement of the trachea and mediastinum, impaired venous return, and severe respiratory distress. Emergent decompression is necessary, although tension pneumothorax is rare in PSP.

Clinical Presentation

Symptoms

PSP: Sudden onset of symptoms, often without an identifiable trigger. Common presentations include:

Chest pain (90% of cases), typically sharp or pleuritic and localized to the affected side.

Dyspnea, reported in 80% of cases but often mild.

SSP: Symptoms, especially dyspnea, tend to be more severe and disproportionate to pneumothorax size due to underlying lung pathology.

Signs

Physical findings may be subtle and include:

Diminished or absent breath sounds on the affected side.

Hyper-resonance to percussion.

Reduced chest wall movement.
Severe cases, particularly tension pneumothorax, may present with cyanosis, tachycardia, hypotension, tracheal deviation, and distended neck veins.

Diagnostic Considerations

Imaging

1. Chest X-ray (CXR): A posteroanterior (PA) view is the primary diagnostic tool. Findings include a visible pleural line, absence of pulmonary markings, and hyperlucency. In trauma patients, a supine CXR may show subtle signs like the deep sulcus sign.

2. Computed Tomography (CT): Considered the gold standard for diagnosis, CT scans differentiate pneumothorax from bullae and assess underlying lung abnormalities.

3. Ultrasound: Increasingly employed, especially in critical care, to identify absent lung sliding and comet-tail artifacts.

Laboratory

Arterial blood gas analysis may be necessary for hypoxic or critically ill patients to evaluate oxygenation.

Treatment

General Principles

Management varies based on symptom severity, pneumothorax size, and patient-specific factors:

Supplemental oxygen accelerates air reabsorption by reducing nitrogen pressure gradients.

Emergency decompression is required for tension pneumothorax, often performed using a small-bore catheter or finger thoracostomy.

Conservative Management

Patients with minimal symptoms and small pneumothoraces may be managed without invasive interventions. Follow-up chest imaging ensures resolution.

Invasive Interventions

1. Simple Aspiration: First-line for symptomatic pneumothorax without significant comorbidities.

2. Chest Tube Drainage: Indicated for large or refractory pneumothoraces, secondary causes, or traumatic injuries.

Emerging evidence supports less invasive approaches for select cases, with ongoing trials aiming to refine guidelines.

Conclusion

Pneumothorax management requires a nuanced approach tailored to etiology, severity, and patient characteristics. While many cases resolve spontaneously, prompt recognition and treatment of complications such as tension pneumothorax are critical for favorable outcomes.

References

1. Bintcliffe, O. J., Hallifax, R. J., Edey, A., et al. (2015). Revisiting the approach to spontaneous pneumothorax management. The Lancet Respiratory Medicine, 3(7), 578–588.

2. MacDuff, A., Arnold, T., & Harvey, J. (2010). British Thoracic Society guidelines for the management of spontaneous pneumothorax: Standards of Care Committee report. Thorax, 62, 18–31.

3. Therapeutic Guidelines: Respiratory (5th ed.). (2015). Melbourne: Therapeutic Guidelines Limited.

4. Baumann, M. H., Strange, C., Heffner, J. E., et al. (2001). American College of Chest Physicians consensus on spontaneous pneumothorax management: A Delphi statement. Chest, 119(2), 590–602.

Chapter 8
Pleural effusion

Key points

1. In most cases, a posteroanterior and lateral chest radiograph is sufficient to confirm and pinpoint the presence of a pleural effusion. For smaller effusions, ultrasound, lateral decubitus radiographs, and computed tomography (CT) scans offer higher diagnostic sensitivity and accuracy.

2. The primary approach to identifying the cause of a pleural effusion is through pleural fluid analysis, which provides critical diagnostic insights.

3. For both diagnostic and therapeutic fluid removal, ultrasound-guided thoracentesis is the preferred and most effective technique.

4. Management strategies depend on the underlying condition. When large pleural effusions cause cardiorespiratory compromise, fluid aspiration is necessary to alleviate symptoms.

5. Transudative effusions typically resolve with treatment directed at the underlying medical issue. In contrast, exudative effusions often require additional diagnostic evaluations and targeted therapeutic interventions.

Introduction

Pleural effusion refers to the abnormal accumulation of fluid within the pleural space, which typically arises due to a disruption in the homeostatic mechanisms regulating pleural fluid balance. While massive pleural effusions can lead to significant cardiorespiratory compromise requiring prompt intervention, many cases present with minimal or no symptoms. In such asymptomatic or minimally symptomatic cases, the primary objective in emergency settings is to identify the underlying cause to guide appropriate treatment. This process involves a comprehensive history, physical examination, and targeted investigations, such as chest X-rays (CXR), thoracic ultrasound, pleural fluid analysis, and, in selected cases, biopsies obtained during thoracentesis. Advanced diagnostic tools like bronchoscopy and thoracoscopy are typically reserved for cases where standard evaluations fail to identify the etiology.

Pathogenesis and Pathophysiology

The pleural cavity is a potential space between the visceral and parietal pleura, lined with mesothelial cells and containing approximately 0.25 mL/kg of low-protein fluid under normal conditions. Fluid movement within this cavity is regulated by capillary pressure, plasma oncotic pressure, and capillary permeability, in accordance with Starling's law. Most pleural fluid is absorbed through pleuro-lymphatic connections, aided by respiratory muscle contractions and intrinsic lymphatic vessel activity. The pleural fluid's production rate is generally balanced by its absorptive capacity, which can exceed normal production by 10-20 times. However, disruptions in these mechanisms result in pleural effusions, which can be categorized into three main groups:

1. Transudative Effusions: Caused by alterations in hydrostatic or osmotic pressure gradients.

2. Exudative Effusions: Resulting from inflammation or loss of semipermeable membrane integrity, leading to protein-rich fluid accumulation.

3. Lymphatic Obstruction: Impeding drainage, often resulting in transudative effusions.

Etiology

Pleural effusions are broadly classified as transudates or exudates based on their underlying causes.

Transudative Causes:

Common Examples: Congestive heart failure, cirrhosis, nephrotic syndrome, hypoalbuminemia, and peritoneal dialysis.

Uncommon Causes: Superior vena cava obstruction, urinothorax, or cerebrospinal fluid leaks.

Exudative Causes:

Infectious Etiologies: Pneumonia, tuberculosis, fungal infections, or empyema.

Malignancies: Carcinomas, lymphomas, and mesotheliomas.

Inflammatory Disorders: Rheumatoid pleurisy, lupus pleuritis, and sarcoidosis.

Trauma and Iatrogenic Factors: Post-thoracic surgery, central venous catheter migration, or drug-induced pleural reactions.

Further subclassification is guided by diagnostic findings, including imaging and pleural fluid analysis.

Classification Using Light's Criteria

The differentiation between transudates and exudates relies on Light's criteria, which compare pleural fluid biochemistry to serum values. A pleural effusion is categorized as an exudate if any of the following is true:

LDH Ratio: Pleural fluid lactate dehydrogenase (LDH) to serum LDH > 0.6.

LDH Level: Pleural fluid LDH exceeds two-thirds of the upper limit of normal for serum LDH.

Protein Ratio: Pleural fluid protein to serum protein > 0.5.

For confirmed exudates, additional investigations are essential to establish the specific etiology.

Clinical Presentation and Evaluation

History and Symptoms:

A detailed patient history often provides vital clues about the effusion's cause. Key aspects include:

Symptom onset, progression, and severity.

Indicators of common causes like heart failure, infection, or malignancy.

Relevant exposures (e.g., tuberculosis, asbestos), medications, or prior surgeries.

Symptoms such as dyspnea are the most common, while chest pain may suggest malignancy, pleural inflammation, or pulmonary embolism. Systemic symptoms (e.g., fever, weight loss) may indicate underlying infections or malignancy.

Physical Examination:

Smaller effusions (<300 mL) may not produce overt physical signs. Larger effusions often present with:

Respiratory Changes: Dyspnea, hypoxemia, reduced chest expansion, or mediastinal shift.

Auscultation Findings: Diminished or absent breath sounds, bronchial breathing above the effusion, or pleural rub.

Percussion: Stony dullness on the affected side.

Diagnostic Investigations

Imaging:

Chest X-ray (CXR): Provides crucial information, including effusion size and localization. Larger effusions are identified by opacity and the meniscus sign, while smaller or loculated effusions may require additional views.

Ultrasound: Superior to CXR in detecting smaller effusions and identifying loculations, pleural thickening, or malignancy.

Computed Tomography (CT): Valuable for detecting subtle effusions and underlying pathologies.

Thoracentesis:

Diagnostic thoracentesis is indispensable when the etiology is unclear. Under ultrasound guidance, pleural fluid is aspirated for:

Biochemical Analysis: LDH, protein, glucose, and pH levels.

Microbiological Testing: Cultures for bacterial, fungal, or mycobacterial organisms.

Cytology: Especially critical for suspected malignancies.

Additional Tests:

Tuberculosis Markers: Acid-fast bacilli and adenosine deaminase levels.

Triglycerides/Cholesterol: For suspected chylothorax or pseudochylothorax.

Amylase: For pancreatic or esophageal etiologies.

Conclusion

The management of pleural effusion necessitates a systematic approach, beginning with a detailed clinical assessment and progressing to targeted investigations. Prompt differentiation between transudative and exudative effusions using Light's criteria is fundamental in guiding further diagnostics and treatment. Advanced imaging and fluid analysis are pivotal in identifying the underlying pathology, ensuring timely and effective management.

References

1. Bhatnagar R, Maskell N. The modern diagnosis and management of pleural effusions. BMJ. 2015;351:h4520.

2. Davies HE, Davies RJ, Davies CW, and the BTS Pleural Disease Guideline Group. Management of pleural infection in adults: British Thoracic Society pleural disease guideline 2010. Thorax. 2010;65(Suppl. 2):ii41–ii53.

3. Havelock T, Teoh R, Laws D, Gleeson F, and the BTS Pleural Disease Guideline Group. Pleural procedures and thoracic ultrasound: British Thoracic Society pleural disease guideline 2010. Thorax. 2010;65(Suppl. 2):ii61–ii76.

4. Hooper C, Lee YC, Maskell N, and the BTS Pleural Guideline Group. Investigation of a unilateral pleural effusion in adults: British Thoracic Society pleural disease guideline 2010. Thorax. 2010;65(Suppl. 2):ii4–ii17.

5. Light RW. Clinical practice: Pleural effusion. N Engl J Med. 2002;346(25):1971–1977.

6. McClune J, Cardenas-Garcia J. Ultrasound guidance for thoracic procedures. Curr Pulmonol Rep. 2017;6(3):187–194.

7. Porcel JM, Light RW. Diagnostic approach to pleural effusion in adults. Am Fam Physician. 2006;73:1211–1220.

8. Rahul B, Nick M. The modern diagnosis and management of pleural effusions. BMJ. 2015;351:h4520.

9. Roberts ME, Neville E, Berrisford RG, Antunes G, Ali NJ, and the BTS Pleural Disease Guideline Group. Management of malignant pleural effusion: British Thoracic Society pleural disease guideline 2010. Thorax. 2010;65(Suppl. 2):ii32–ii40.

10. Wong CL, Holroyd-Leduc J, Straus SE. Does this patient have a pleural effusion? JAMA. 2009;301:309–317.

Chapter 9
Haemoptysis

Key Points

1. Most patients presenting with haemoptysis can be safely evaluated and treated in an outpatient setting.

2. Differentiating haemoptysis from haematemesis or bleeding originating from the upper airway is crucial for appropriate management.

3. A normal chest X-ray does not exclude significant pathology, as it may appear normal in 30% of haemoptysis cases and can fail to detect 25% of malignancies.

4. High-resolution computed tomography (HRCT) is the preferred diagnostic tool when a

chest X-ray does not reveal the cause of bleeding.

5. Bronchoscopy is particularly valuable for identifying lesions within the bronchial tree that may be causing haemoptysis.

6. In approximately 50% of haemoptysis cases, no identifiable cause is determined despite thorough evaluation.

7. Managing massive haemoptysis requires prioritizing ventilation, oxygenation, circulatory stability, and prompt identification and treatment of the bleeding source.

8. For patients requiring intubation, selecting the appropriate endotracheal tube and determining its optimal placement pose significant challenges.

9. Emergency embolization of bleeding vessels can temporarily halt hemorrhage, providing

critical time for patient stabilization before definitive surgical intervention.

Introduction

Haemoptysis, defined as the expectoration of blood originating from the lungs or tracheobronchial tree, is a clinical symptom that varies in severity. Most patients report small amounts of blood mixed with sputum or saliva and can be managed in outpatient settings. However, a minority present with massive haemoptysis, a life-threatening condition characterized by significant respiratory and circulatory compromise. These critical cases demand immediate and skilled intervention to secure the airway and maintain circulation, as rapid asphyxiation or exsanguination can occur. Even a minor blood clot can obstruct ventilation as effectively as a substantial bleed that inundates an entire lung.

Aetiology

Haemoptysis has numerous potential causes, which are summarized in Table 6.8.1. In up to 50% of cases, no identifiable cause is found.

Clinical Features

Approximately 95% of patients with haemoptysis do not present with life-threatening bleeding. Massive haemoptysis, which poses an immediate threat to life, is typically due to respiratory compromise caused by airway obstruction or ventilatory impairment with as little as 200 mL of blood.

Patients often confuse haemoptysis with haematemesis, requiring careful differentiation. Haemoptysis typically involves bright red, frothy, alkaline blood expelled by coughing, while gastrointestinal bleeding appears darker, may contain food particles, and is acidic. Haemoptysis must also be distinguished from nasopharyngeal bleeding, such as epistaxis.

A thorough history and physical examination should focus on:

Assessing airway obstruction and cardiorespiratory compromise.

Identifying symptoms associated with infections, neoplasms, tuberculosis (TB), vasculitis, or other chronic or acute respiratory conditions.

Considering recent procedures, anticoagulation therapy, TB exposure, foreign bodies, or past medical history of vasculitis.

Diagnostic Investigations

Chest X-Ray

A chest x-ray is the initial diagnostic modality and may reveal new alveolar opacities that localize bleeding. Chronic lung diseases, infections, masses, cavitations, or cardiopulmonary abnormalities may also be identified. However, chest x-rays fail to detect tumors in 25% of bleeding cases.

Computed Tomography (CT)

If a chest x-ray is inconclusive, high-resolution CT (HRCT) can provide detailed pulmonary imaging. HRCT identifies the source of haemoptysis in over 65% of cases and is particularly effective in diagnosing malignancies. CT pulmonary angiography is valuable for detecting pulmonary embolism or vascular malformations.

Bronchoscopy

With advances in CT imaging, the diagnostic role of bronchoscopy has declined. However, in cases of massive haemoptysis, it is crucial for localizing and treating bleeding lesions. Bronchoscopy also facilitates the collection of sputum or cytological samples for further analysis.

Laboratory Tests and Other Modalities

Sputum Analysis: Universal precautions are essential when suspecting infectious causes like TB.

Blood Work: Complete blood counts, coagulation studies, and assessments of oxygenation (pulse oximetry or venous blood gas analysis) are critical. Blood grouping and cross-matching may be required for massive haemoptysis.

Other Investigations: Nasoendoscopy, biopsy, or advanced imaging like MRI may be warranted if the source of bleeding is suspected to involve the upper airway.

Treatment

Non-Massive Haemoptysis

In mild cases, haemoptysis is often self-limiting and managed by addressing the underlying cause. Outpatient management with antibiotics may suffice, though follow-up is necessary to exclude malignancies.

Massive Haemoptysis

This severe condition, accounting for less than 2% of haemoptysis cases, has a mortality rate exceeding 50%. Tuberculosis, bronchiectasis, infections, and malignancies are common causes.

Management priorities include:

1. Airway, Breathing, Circulation (ABC): Immediate interventions address hypoxia and maintain ventilation. Early consultation with specialists (e.g., respiratory physicians, interventional radiologists, anesthetists, or thoracic surgeons) is vital.

2. Imaging: Rapid acquisition of chest x-ray or HRCT helps localize bleeding.

3. Oxygenation: Oxygen delivery via mask or nasal prongs is initiated, with intubation considered for severe hypoxia.

Advanced Interventions

Intubation

Securing the airway is challenging due to limited visibility and oxygen reserves. Options include single-lumen endotracheal tubes (ETTs), double-lumen ETTs, or selective lung intubation. Double-lumen ETTs allow independent ventilation and bleeding control but require advanced expertise.

Circulation and Hemostasis

Blood transfusion and correction of coagulopathies are essential. Tranexamic acid may temporarily reduce bleeding, though evidence is limited.

Interventional Radiology

Bronchial artery embolization is a key therapeutic option, achieving immediate success in 70–99% of cases. While rebleeding is possible, this technique often stabilizes patients sufficiently for surgical interventions.

Bronchoscopy

Rigid bronchoscopy enables effective blood clearance and improved ventilation during massive haemoptysis. Flexible bronchoscopes are better suited for smaller airways but have limited suctioning capacity.

Surgical Management

Surgical resection is controversial but may be necessary for recurrent or intractable bleeding. Surgery is typically reserved for stable patients or cases involving lesions such as vascular malformations.

Additional Measures

Adjunctive therapies include endobronchial balloon tamponade, topical adrenaline, or antifungal agents for mycetoma-related haemoptysis. Conservative management may involve airway suctioning and supportive care.

Controversies

Optimal patient positioning during massive haemoptysis.

Preferred method of intubation in acute settings.

Choice between rigid and flexible bronchoscopy.

Role and timing of tranexamic acid administration.

Balancing conservative and operative management strategies.

Conclusion

Effective management of haemoptysis requires an accurate diagnosis, careful differentiation of causes, and a tailored approach to treatment, particularly in life-threatening cases. Integrating diagnostic tools, therapeutic interventions, and multidisciplinary expertise is essential for optimal outcomes.

References

1. Ittrich H, Bockhorn M, Klose H, Simon M. Diagnosis and management of hemoptysis. Dtsch Arztebl Int. 2017;114(21):371–381.

2. Herth F, Ernst A, Becker HD. Long-term prognosis and lung cancer risk in patients with idiopathic hemoptysis. Chest. 2001;120(5):1592–1594.

3. Larici AR, Franchi P, Occhipinti M, et al. Approaches to diagnosing and treating hemoptysis. Diagn Interv Radiol. 2014;20(4):299–309.

4. Nielsen K, Gottlieb M, Colella S, et al. The utility of bronchoscopy alongside computed tomography in evaluating patients with hemoptysis. Eur Clin Resp J. 2016;3(1):31802.

5. Jean-Baptiste E. Assessment and management strategies for massive hemoptysis. Crit Care Med. 2000;28(5):1642–1647.

6. Moen CA, Burrell A, Dunning J. Efficacy of tranexamic acid in controlling hemoptysis. Interact Cardiovasc Thorac Surg. 2013;17(6):991–994.

7. Panda A, Bhalla AS, Goyal A. The role of bronchial artery embolization in hemoptysis: A systematic review. Diagn Interv Radiol. 2017;23(4):307–317.